THE ABSENT BODY

THE ABSENT BODY

DREW LEDER

THE UNIVERSITY OF CHICAGO PRESS
CHICAGO AND LONDON

The University of Chicago Press, Chicago 60637
The University of Chicago Press, Ltd., London
© 1990 by The University of Chicago
All rights reserved. Published 1990
Printed and bound by CPI Group (UK) Ltd,
Croydon, CR0 4YY

99 98 97 96 95   5 4 3

Library of Congress Cataloging-in-Publication Data

Leder. Drew.
  The absent body / Drew Leder.
    p. cm.
  Includes bibliographical references.
  ISBN 0–226–46999–9 —ISBN 0–226–47000–8 (pbk.)
  1. Body, Human (Philosophy)   2. Mind and body.   3. Dualism.
I. Title.
B105.B64L43   1990
128'.3—dc20   89–49193
                                                            CIP

⊗ The paper used in this publication meets the minimum
requirements of the American National Standard for Information
Sciences–Permanence of Paper for Printed Library Materials,
ANSI Z39.48–1984.

To my family:
my parents, Harold and Gertrude,
and my brother, Scott

The University of Chicago Press, Chicago 60637
The University of Chicago Press, Ltd., London
© 1990 by The University of Chicago
All rights reserved. Published 1990
Printed in the United States of America
16 15 14 13 12 11 10 09 08 07   4 5 6 7 8

ISBN-13: 978-0-226-47000-9 (paper)
ISBN-10: 0-226-47000-8 (paper)

Library of Congress Cataloging-in-Publication Data

Leder, Drew.
    The absent body / Drew Leder.
        p.   cm.
    Includes bibliographical references.
    ISBN 0-226-46999-9—ISBN 0-226-47000-8 (pbk.)
    1. Body, Human (Philosophy).   2. Mind and body.   3. Dualism.
I. Title.
B105.B64L43   1990
128'.3—dc20   89-49193
                                                            CIP

♾ The paper used in this publication meets the minimum
requirements of the American National Standard for Information
Sciences—Permanence of Paper for Printed Library Materials,
ANSI Z39.48-1992.

Contents

Acknowledgments

Through God's grace, I have been assisted by many individuals and institutions during the preparation of this manuscript. This assistance has taken several forms including textual criticism, personal encouragement, organizational support, and inspirational example. In acknowledging my debt of gratitude it is difficult to know where to begin and leave off.

But not too difficult; I would first like to thank Ed Casey. It is not simply that this manuscript has benefitted from his careful critique. More generally, my turn to the profession of philosophy might never have happened except through his encouragement. I feel most lucky to have found such a friend and mentor.

Many others have contributed to this work in ways now impossible to unravel. Mary Rawlinson, Don Ihde, and Michael Schwartz all read the manuscript at its various stages and provided helpful suggestions. Carol Fessler's careful and literate proofreading was invaluable. Discussions with David Abram and David Strong on the body, technology, and ecology greatly stimulated my thinking. I was inspired not only by the ideas of such individuals but their sense of the raw excitement, the sheer *importance,* of philosophy. Here too I think of Ron Scapp.

A different sort of assistance came from D. R. Gilroy, Jr. and members of the Recovery Alliance, Inc. Their help in opening spiritual doors to a recalcitrant seeker led to the ideas embedded in my final chapter. The conceptual structure needed to develop these ideas evolved from discussions with Robert Neville; his excitement concerning Neo-Confucianism proved infectious.

On a personal level, I am indebted to Phyllis, Robert, and Betsy McLane for all the warmth and support they have provided. As for institutional support, I have been twice blessed; a generous fellowship from the State University of New York at Stony Brook and a sabbatical leave granted through The Loyola College Center for the Humanities both provided crucial time for pursuing my research.

Finally, I wish to thank my wife, Janice McLane. She has been a constant source of loving encouragement, a voice of reason amidst the madness of writing, and an intellectual colleague who has tested my thinking and supplemented it with new perspectives. Such is the privilege of having for a wife such a good friend *and* a fellow philosopher.

I would like to thank Alfred A. Knopf, Inc. and Andre Deutsch Ltd. for permission to reprint the poem "Pain," by John Updike, from *Facing*

Nature, © 1985 by John Updike. The untitled poem #650 by Emily Dickinson has been reprinted by permission of the publishers and the Trustees of Amherst College from *The Poems of Emily Dickinson,* edited by Thomas H. Johnson, Cambridge, MA: The Belknap Press of Harvard University Press, copyright 1951, © 1955, 1979, 1983 by the President and Fellows of Harvard College.

Introduction

Human experience is incarnated. I receive the surrounding world through my eyes, my ears, my hands. The structure of my perceptual organs shapes that which I apprehend. And it is via bodily means that I am capable of responding. My legs carry me toward a desired goal seen across the distance. My hands reach out to take up tools, reconstructing the natural surroundings into an abode uniquely suited to my body. My actions are motivated by emotions, needs, desires, that well up from a corporeal self. Relations with others are based upon our mutuality of gaze and touch, our speech, our resonances of feeling and perspective. From the most visceral of cravings to the loftiest of artistic achievements, the body plays its formative role.

Yet this bodily presence is of a highly paradoxical nature. While in one sense the body is the most abiding and inescapable presence in our lives, it is also essentially characterized by absence. That is, one's own body is rarely the thematic object of experience. When reading a book or lost in thought, my own bodily state may be the farthest thing from my awareness. I experientially dwell in a world of ideas, paying little heed to my physical sensations or posture. Nor is this forgetfulness restricted to moments of higher-level cognition. I may be engaged in a fierce sport, muscles flexed and responsive to the slightest movements of my opponent. Yet it is precisely upon this opponent, this game, that my attention dwells, not on my own embodiment.

We find this same absence recapitulated when we think according to specific regions of the body. For example, a psychological experiment has shown that nine out of ten people are incapable of picking out a photograph of their own hands from a small series of such pictures.[1] That organ with which I perform my labor, eat my food, caress my loved ones, yet remains a stranger to me. This strangeness is even more pronounced in the case of the internal organs. I would surely be unable to recognize the look of my own heart, though my very life depends upon its functions.

This work will be primarily devoted to exploring this corporeal absence. I will seek to elucidate its essential structures and trace out its philosophical implications. That is, I will try to answer the question of why the body, as a ground of experience, yet tends to recede from direct experience. However, this seemingly simple question will yield a complex and diverse set of answers. This follows from the diversity of the

1

body itself. Far from being a homogenous thing, the body is a complex harmony of different regions, each operating according to indigenous principles and incorporating different parts of the world into its space. Hence, the modes of absence that characterize different bodily parts and activities will themselves differ. The invisibility of the eye within its own visual field, the diaphanous embodiment of language, the inaccessibility of the visceral organs: these all exhibit their own principles of absence, which can only be teased apart by a careful investigation.

But why conduct such an investigation? The first and most obvious reason lies in its intrinsic phenomenological significance. An exploration of such absences, far from being a peripheral matter, will serve to reveal the essential structures of embodiment. The import of this topic has already been suggested by developments in twentieth-century Continental philosophy. On the one hand, the phenomenological centrality of the body is elucidated in the works of Husserl, Merleau-Ponty, Sartre, Marcel, Straus, Jonas, and a host of others upon whom I will draw. On the other hand, the theme of absence has recently been highlighted both as a development within and a challenge to traditional phenomenological thought. Most famously, Derrida has criticized the "metaphysics of presence," exposing the self-effacements and deferments that lie hidden at the heart of any ideal of pure presence.[2] Sokolowski has clarified the crucial role of absence in the acquisition and use of language.[3] Yet the body has remained but a marginal topic to such authors. Conversely, nowhere in the literature on embodiment is the notion of absence comprehensively explored. The volume which most renders this concept central, Merleau-Ponty's *The Visible and the Invisible*,[4] was sadly truncated by the author's premature death. Merleau-Ponty has exercised a great influence upon my thinking, and my own text, in its inevitably imperfect fashion, has sought to continue his project in certain ways.

In other ways, it seeks to go beyond. Phenomenological studies of embodiment, including those of Merleau-Ponty, have primarily revolved around themes of perception and motility. It is through these modalities that we directly experience and act upon the world. Yet such functions arise within a series of impersonal horizons: the embryonic body prior to birth, the autonomous rhythms of breathing and circulation, the stilled body of sleep, the mystery of the corpse. It is precisely because such bodily states involve various forms of experiential absence that they have tended to be neglected by philosophers of experience. However, until these anonymous bodies are recognized, our self-understanding remains incomplete.

Besides such phenomenological yields, the theme of bodily absence is of no little cultural significance. It has often been observed that modern

Western society is typified by a certain "disembodied" style of life. Our shelters protect us from direct corporeal engagement with the outer world, our relative prosperity alleviating, for many of us, immediate physical need and distress. Via machines we are disinvested of work that once belonged to the muscles. Technologies of rapid communication and transportation allow us to transcend what used to be the natural limits imposed by the body. Operations are mediated by the written word or the computer calculation, where once a living human presence was required. A rising interest in finding ways to "return to the body," whether via exercise, hatha yoga, body therapies, craft-work, or intimacy with nature, is but a reaction to this general trend toward a "decorporealized" existence.

Such social developments can only be understood in relation to the modes of absence inherent in the body. Cultural variations are always played out upon the keyboard of possibilities presented by our corporeal structure. Only because the body has intrinsic tendencies toward self-concealment could such tendencies be exaggerated by linguistic and technological extensions.

Furthermore, far from being indigenous just to modern society, a certain telos toward disembodiment is an abiding strain of Western intellectual history. The Platonic emphasis on the purified soul, the Cartesian focus on the "cogito" experience, pull us toward a vision of self within which an immaterial rationality is central. The body has frequently been relegated to a secondary or oppositional role, while an incorporeal reason is valorized.

This brings me to a further purpose of this study: its import vis-à-vis the history of ideas. To a great extent our culture is still under the sway of the Cartesian paradigm. It is often assumed that this dualist paradigm is shaped by ontological commitments at the expense of attending to lived experience. However, I will argue against this view. I will suggest that experience plays a crucial role in encouraging and supporting Cartesian dualism. Specifically, I refer to experiences of bodily *absence*. Such experiences, as I will later discuss, seem to support the doctrine of an immaterial mind trapped inside an alien body. I am not in sympathy with this dualist portrayal. Yet I seek a phenomenological account of why Cartesian-style dualism would be so persuasive. Only in such a way can we break its conceptual hegemony, while simultaneously reclaiming its experiential truths.

This project of reclamation accounts for the unusual progression of this work. Ordinarily one would clear the ground for a novel discussion of body by criticizing previous historical positions. In my case, argument proceeds in an opposite direction. It is precisely the phenomenology of bodily absence that will provide the tool for understanding previous concepts of self. The original phenomenology must then largely precede the historical rereading.

The first part of this work, comprising the first three chapters, is thus devoted to "Phenomenological Investigations." In chapter 1, I will examine the modes of absence characteristic of the surface of the human body, whose sensorimotor powers open onto the world. As this is the aspect of embodiment upon which phenomenologists have focused, a good part of this chapter, though by no means all, will be devoted to consolidating and extending the work of previous authors. In chapter 2, I will shift attention to the bodily depths. I will explore the way in which the visceral organs, along with certain of the body's temporal modes, recede from personal apprehension and control. The sort of absence involved will be revealed as importantly different from, though intertwined with, that which characterizes the surface body. In chapter 3, I will then define a mode of presence-absence correlative with those previously discussed. Insofar as the body tends to disappear when functioning unproblematically, it often seizes our attention most strongly at times of dysfunction; we then experience the body as the very *absence* of a desired or ordinary state, and as a force that stands opposed to the self. I will discuss examples such as pain, disease, and social breakdown to illustrate this principle.

The second part of this work, entitled "Philosophical Consequences," will then articulate the significance of these findings vis-à-vis the history of ideas. It is, in a sense, the payoff of all that has come before. In chapter 4, I will explore Descartes's account of the immateriality of mind, tracing out its dependence on the modes of bodily disappearance I earlier discussed. In chapter 5, I will address the Cartesian portrayal of body as the negative or oppositional moment within the self. Referring back to the discussions of chapter 3, I will argue that the experiential prominence of the body precisely at times of breakdown and dysfunction helps to foster this negative view.

One of the compelling reasons to challenge Cartesianism has to do with its far-reaching social effects. This hierarchical dualism has been used to subserve projects of oppression directed toward women, animals, nature, and other "Others." In my concluding chapter I thus turn attention to questions of an ethical nature. I address the values that might be associated with the new paradigm of embodiment discussed in this work. Here, I take my cue from a Neo-Confucian notion, adapted for contemporary use: it is the notion that we "form one body" with all things. The body is "absent" only because it is perpetually outside itself, caught up in a multitude of involvements with other people, with nature, with a sacred domain. I thus explore modes of moral, aesthetic, and spiritual communion possible for the embodied self.

Before launching into the main text, it would be useful to say a few preliminary words concerning the concept of body that I will employ. Far from being an unproblematic notion, embodiment has become a focus of phenomenological interest only by virtue of a radical questioning of the previous concepts that have held sway. Since the seventeenth century the body has been primarily identified with its scientific description, i.e., regarded as a material object whose anatomical and functional properties can be characterized according to general scientific law. As such, the human body, while perhaps unusual in its complexity, is taken as essentially no different from any other physical object. In Cartesian terms, it is but a part of *res extensa*.

Merleau-Ponty, drawing upon the work of Husserl, Straus, and others, is the thinker who most systematically challenged this basic presumption. The body as he describes it is never just an object in the world but that very medium whereby our world comes into being.[5] It is via my sensorimotor powers that I encounter a world charged with meaning and organized into significant gestalts. Within this perceptual world the body can itself appear as but another object to be perceived and scientifically described. However, this never exhausts its meaning. The very possibility of objects as we know them, of science, of world, refers us back to that body on the other side of things, the body-as-experiencer. In articulating this dual perspective, philosophers have often utilized the distinction within the German language between *Korper* (physical body) and *Leib* (living body). Cartesianism tends to entrap the human body in the image of *Korper,* treating it as one instance of the general class of physical things. Yet the body understood as *Leib* (or "lived body," as it is commonly translated into English) reveals the deeper significance of corporeality as generative principle.

This notion of lived body provides a potential mode of escape from cognitive habits of dualism deeply entrenched in our culture. Insofar as the body is restricted to its causal-physicalistic description, those aspects of self involving cognition and intentionality are commonly relegated to a substance called "mind." This division of labor between *res extensa* and *res cogitans,* between the scientific and the humanistic domains, is the very basis of Cartesian ontology. Yet this is precisely what the concept of the lived body subverts. If the body as lived structure is a locus of experience, then one need not ascribe this capability to a decorporealized mind. The self is viewed as an integrated being.

In my own work, concerned with the phenomenological critique of Cartesianism, it is particularly important to seek a concept of embodiment that avoids dualistic presumptions. This is why I employ such a broad notion of the lived body, equating it with the embodied self that lives and breathes, perceives and acts, speaks and reasons. Common even in the phenomenological literature are certain partialized conceptions of the lived body that threaten to give rise to new dualisms. For example, we have seen that the notion of the lived body first arose in contradistinction to the body viewed purely as physical entity. However, while of provisional use, if this distinction is overemphasized or ontologized another dualism remains: now not between mind and body per se, but between *Leib* and *Korper*.

This opposition can arise when we identify the lived body solely with the first-person perspective, the body lived-from-within, as opposed to the "object body" seen from without. Indeed, in his discussions of lived embodiment Merleau-Ponty frequently makes use of the term *corps propre* (one's own body),[6] which might suggest a privileging of the first-person point of view. However, as Merleau-Ponty emphasizes especially in his later work, it is intrinsic to lived embodiment to be *both* subject and an object available to external gaze.[7] A Cartesian mind may exhibit metaphysical privacy, but this cannot be true of a visible, situated, fleshly being. There are, in fact, certain bodily profiles, aspects of one's moods and intentions, that are far more available to others than oneself. Hence, while beginning from the first-person perspective, I will have occasion to make frequent reference to the body as it registers in public experience. The very intertwining of self and Other, of body subject and object, will form an ongoing theme in this work.

The notion of the lived body may also be partialized when we ignore the perspective of scientific anatomy and physiology. This presumes that the hard-won battle of freeing *Leib* from *Korper* can only be preserved by a fierce methodological dualism wherein phenomenology remains unsullied by empirical science. Yet, such a dualism is itself the heritage of a Cartesian ontology; the separation of *res cogitans* and *res extensa* mandated separate discourses for the intentional and the physical spheres. This division is once again subverted by the move to lived embodiment. To be a lived body is always also to be a physical body with bones and tendons, nerves and sinews, all of which can be scientifically characterized. These are not two different bodies. *Korper* is itself an aspect of *Leib*, one manner in which the lived body shows itself.

When the scientific account is taken as the only correct and foundational metaphysics we do fall into a pernicious scientism. But once relativized within a broader phenomenological reading, scientific references need not be reductionistic; they can open up a rich experiential domain. For science itself arises out of lived experience, albeit of a specialized sort. The scientific account emphasizes the body as experienced from a third-person rather than a first-person perspective. Moreover, the scientist tends to perceive objects through highly developed technologies and conceptual strategies uncommon to the ordinary life-world.[8] The scientific account is thus radically incomplete for our philosophical purposes. All the other perceptual perspectives it has systematically expunged must be recalled and revalorized. Yet it would be a mistake to then expunge from our view the specialized experiences of the scientist. Such experiences reveal aspects of corporeality unavailable to ordinary vision and clarify the structural correlates to intentional capabilities. I will thus at certain points utilize the findings of science as a clue to the nature of lived embodiment. My own interest in such matters has been stimulated by a training in medicine as well as philosophy. I take it that this disciplinary cross-fertilization is not merely permitted but encouraged by the notion of the lived body, for this concept challenges traditional dualisms, both ontological and methodological in form.

There remains one other way in which the notion of the lived body has been partialized. Within phenomenology the lived body has often been identified primarily with one's immediate sensorimotor grasp upon the world, as contrasted with faculties of abstract cognition. This contrast, as that between *Leib* and *Korper,* was crucial at a certain point in clearing the ground and permitting the recognition of a range of phenomena. As Merleau-Ponty elucidated, it is our lived body itself, not an intellectual mind, that first perceives objects, knows its way around a room, senses the sadness in another's face. Such sensorimotor abilities are not merely a form of conception; they do not depend on explicit judgments, categories, or rules. Rather, they exhibit a more primordial intentionality, which must be accorded its own logic. However, to identify the lived body solely with this sensorimotor level to the exclusion of "higher" forms of cognition obscures the larger significance of what has been revealed. As Merleau-Ponty suggests, abstract cognition itself may sublimate but never fully escapes its inherence in a perceiving, acting body.[9] I will thus examine the lived body as the seat of intellectual thought, no less than that of a prethematic sensory grasp. This is an important theme in a work that seeks to explicate the bodily roots of Cartesian dualism.

To summarize, the notion of lived body here employed refers to the embodied person witnessed from the third-person and first-person perspective alike, articulated by science as well as the life-world gaze, including intellectual cognition along with visceral and sensorimotor capacities. To use the term "lived body" (or simply "body" for short) in such a comprehensive fashion may seem misleading and reductionistic.

However, my goal is not in any way to impoverish our sense of humanity, as if the self were "just" a body. Rather, it is to progressively enrich our notion of the body by showing its influence throughout the human domain.

Nor, to add a personal note, is my intent to deny a spiritual dimension of life. My attack upon the "immateriality" of reason may seem a categorical denial that there exists within us any core that communicates with a universal or divine principle. Yet this is not at all my desire or my own belief. On the contrary, I think that to equate reason with this divine principle truncates spiritual inquiry. It is part and parcel of a modern zeitgeist wherein human rationality is worshipped as the guiding principle of our world. The unhappy results of this blind faith in the intellect and its scientific and technological powers is everywhere evident in contemporary society.

In Cartesianism, the human mind is viewed as an island of awareness afloat in a vast sea of insensate matter. The notion of the lived body makes room for a more inclusive sense of spirit—one immanent throughout the physical world and expressing itself at all levels of nature, as in a Whiteheadian or animistic ontology. Room is thus made for a sense of spirit-in-immanence through deflating the hubris of rational mind. Yet the importance of this deflation is recognized equally by spiritual traditions that adhere to a more transcendent ideal. Many religions have emphasized the import of differentiating between the eternal Self (Soul, Atman, Buddha Nature) and the mind, that collection of chattering thoughts, desires, dispositions, and intellectual powers that go to make up the personal ego. From the perspective of the mystic, the true Self lies beyond not simply the body but this individualized mentality. To identify with the latter is to deepen the illusion of the separated self, which blocks the realization of interconnection.

In my own belief there is a divine source of awareness of which the individual lived body partakes, but which it does not exhaust. However, my intent is not to argue such a case. Such metaphysical concerns lie beyond the scope of this work, which is, after all, a piece of phenomenology. My point is simply that a recognition of lived embodiment does not foreclose such questions or interpretive paths. On the contrary, shattering the rigid model of Cartesianism clears the way for expanded ontologies.

I
PHENOMENOLOGICAL
INVESTIGATIONS

1

The Ecstatic Body

What ["consciousness"] does not see it does not see for reasons of principle, it is because it is consciousness that it does not see. *What* it does not see is what in it prepares the vision of the rest (as the retina is blind at the point where the fibers that will permit the vision spread out into it). *What* it does not see is what makes it see, is its tie to Being, is its corporeity, are the existentials by which the world becomes visible, is the flesh wherein the *ob*ject is born.

Maurice Merleau-Ponty, *The Visible and the Invisible,* Working Notes, May 1960

It is through the bodily surface that I first engage the world. Only because my eyes and ears lie on the surface of my body are they capable of disclosing the events taking place around me. My hands, in order to explore and work upon the world, must extend outward from my corporeal "extremities." My expressive face can form a medium of communication only because it is available to the Other's gaze. No organ concealed in the hidden depths of the body could actualize intersubjectivity in this way. It is thus necessary that our perceptual, motor, and communicative powers cluster at or near the body surface. The surface is where self meets what is other than self.

In this first chapter I will focus exclusively upon the sensorimotor surface of the body, seeking the structural principles that govern its operation. Methodologically, I will also begin on the surface; that is, I will commence with an artificially simplified analysis, only gradually working my way to more in-depth models. An examination of the visual field considered in isolation will form my initial point of entry.

Perception

Out on a country walk, I pause to lean against a picket fence. My attention is drawn to a large sycamore that dominates the surrounding countryside. This tree becomes the central focus of my visual field. However, it is always placed within and articulated against a background of which I am peripherally aware—the sloping, grassy hill upon which the tree grows, the blue sky mottled with clouds. This structure of figure-ground complementarity which typifies any perceptual field has been extensively investigated by Gestalt psychologists and will not be discussed at length here. Instead, I will concentrate upon the

11

role of the body vis-à-vis this field. I note that my own body may make an appearance within the visual panorama. Out of the corner of my eye I catch sight of my foot extending between the fence posts, my elbow jutting out. I can shift my head to gaze directly upon these. Regions of my body may thus present themselves as part of the background or the central focus of my visual field.

However, this is not the case for the entirety of my body. Barring for the moment the question of mirrors, I find I cannot gaze upon large portions of my back side, especially from the waist up. Furthermore, I cannot see, with the exception of a protruding tongue or nose, most of my face. As Merleau-Ponty writes, "my body as given to me by sight is broken at the height of the shoulders and terminates in a tactile-muscular object."[1] Nor can I rectify this deficiency by simply shifting position to get a better view. While this strategy works with external objects, the body naturally limits attempts to get a new angle upon it. Wherever I go to gaze at it, it comes with me as itself the source of the gaze.[2]

I find that the disappearance of bodily regions is directly related to their proximity to this source. The head is absent insofar as it immediately surrounds and underlies the eyes such that the eyes cannot achieve a perspective upon it. As I approach the center point and origin of vision I lapse into an invisibility no less certain than that which takes hold of objects increasingly distant. My eyes themselves never appear within their visual field except indirectly via reflective surfaces. It is not that I perceive a sort of gap or darkness where my eyes should be; the visual field simply begins and ends in front of them. As the origin of vision, the eyes are also its terminus.

Yet, while I do not directly see these eyes, they maintain a pervasive presence in the experienced world. The objects I do see refer back to my eyes in a series of implicit modes. I know that the very existence of this visual spectacle rests upon my power of sight. Furthermore, that place from which sight originates constitutes an orientational center for the optical field.[3] Everything stands to the right or left of my eyes, above or below, near or far from them, and it is in this way that things take up a determinate relation to one another. The location of my eyes floods throughout the visual world, organizing and giving it sense as the vanishing point organizes every brushstroke of a Renaissance painting. My eyes themselves are the prototype of this vanishing point, an implicit omnipresence nowhere to be seen.

This absence is intrinsic to the perspectival nature of embodiment. As Merleau-Ponty writes, "to be situated within a certain point of view necessarily involves not seeing that point of view itself."[4] To be a perspectival being also means that things can only present themselves from a particular angle and through a limited set of profiles. There will necessarily be aspects of any perceptual object, hidden sides, concealed depths, that elude one's gaze. The absence that haunts the perceived world is thus correlative with that of the perceiver.[5] Moreover, this absence is not simply a deficit but a constitutive principle of the real. The inexhaustible depth of the perceptual object, ever promising more than I now see, is precisely what lends it the texture of reality, distinguishing it from the flat image or hallucination.

Thus, we can understand neither the origin, orientation, nor texture of the perceptual field without reference to the absent presence of the perceiving body. This constitutes the necessary supplement to the Gestaltist figure-background description of perception. As Merleau-Ponty writes:

> one's own body is the third term, always tacitly understood, in the figure-background structure, and every figure stands out against the double horizon of external and bodily space.[6]

Referring, as does Merleau-Ponty, to the body as part of a double horizon risks obscuring a crucial divergence between two sorts of phenomena. The external visual horizon that stretches behind the thematized figure retains a vague and peripheral visibility even while fading into indistinctness. My eyes are more definitively invisible, showing nowhere in my field of vision. And whereas the horizon fades by virtue of its indefinite stretch, becoming imperceptible as it expands behind and away from the figure, the converse is true of my own eyes. It is as space gathers itself together, converging from all angles into a nodal point, that a visual terminus is reached.

Thus, in place of the term *horizon,* I will utilize the Husserlian notion of the *nullpoint (Nullpunkt)*.[7] (My use of this term is provisional, for I will later come to criticize it in certain ways.) In *Ideas 2,* Husserl observes that my lived body (*Leib*) always constitutes a nullpoint in the world I inhabit. No matter where I physically move, and even in the midst of motion, my body retains the status of an absolute "here" around which all "theres" are arrayed. In his work on lived embodiment Husserl had not fully broken with objectivist characterizations.[8] The "nullity" of the nullpoint suggests geometrical terminology wherein the center of any Cartesian coordinate system is defined as zero. Yet this term also expresses the experiential paradox hitherto discussed. Precisely as the center point from which the perceptual field radiates, the perceptual organ remains an absence or nullity in the midst of the perceived.

Admittedly, this absence can be partially circumvented. I can see my eyes and face via the use of mirrors and other reflective surfaces. Yet as Husserl, Sartre, and Merleau-Ponty have all pointed out, there is a crucial incompleteness to the mirror phenomenon. When I catch sight of my eyes in a mirror what I see are constituted objects in the world. I can take note of their color and shape but, as Sartre notes, "I cannot 'see the seeing'; that is, I can not apprehend it in the process of revealing an aspect of the world to me."[9] The eyes-as-seen intertwine, but never phenomenologically coincide, with the eyes as the agent of sight,[10] which involves that invisible power that gives rise to and orients the visual world. Within the world thus disclosed my eyes-as-seen can secondarily appear. Yet these lidded green orbs strangely beg the question. In Merleau-Ponty's words:

> when I try to fill this void by recourse to the image in the mirror, it refers me back to an original of the body which is not out there among things, but in my own province, on this side of all things seen.[11]

The visible eyes cannot fill up or nullify vision's nullpoint.

The body need not rely on external mirrors in order to reflect but can turn its own powers back upon itself, utilizing one organ to examine another. Yet once again, a noncoincidence reigns between perceiver and perceived. This can be illustrated with an example that has played a crucial role in phenomenological discussion of the body from the early Husserl[12] to the late Merleau-Ponty:[13] that of one hand touching another. When my right hand reaches out to touch, I "exist" it as a power of sensing. I do not attend to the hand as physical thing but employ it as that through which I explore the world. Yet I can also reach out with my left hand to touch the right. Can I not then capture at one and the same moment the right hand as touching and touched, thereby filling in the nullpoint, uniting the "subject body" and the "object body"? Not exactly. A careful examination shows that insofar as one attends to the right hand as an object under the touch of the left, one no longer experiences the right hand qua the power of touching. Within the tactile field reorganized around the left hand, the right hand now makes its appearance as a soft fleshy mass. But I cannot "touch it touching" anymore than I could "see the seeing." As soon as the right hand recaptures its power, becoming that with which I feel and explore, it disappears to a degree as thematic object. Within touch, no less than vision, the phenomenon of the nullpoint occurs.

It is thus possible to state a general principle: insofar as I perceive through an organ, it necessarily recedes from the perceptual field it discloses. I do not smell my nasal tissue, hear my ear, or taste my taste buds but perceive with and through such organs. This is not to deny the significant distinctions between sense modalities. Erwin Straus, for example, has explored the very different experiences of spatiality, temporality, and self-object relations that characterize the various senses.[14] Similarly, each mode of sensing involves a different apprehension of one's embodiment. In a distance-sense like sight, one has little or no experience of physical effort or forceful interaction with the perceived object.[15] As such, one's corporeality recedes more thoroughly than in touch, whose reciprocity and feeling of impact calls one back to the copresence of the body with its object. In taste, the experience of world and body is perhaps most closely interwoven; the act of perceiving involves the literal incorporation of the perceived.

Yet for all that distinguishes them, the senses share an essential structure.[16] They all open up upon a world, that which Straus terms the *Allon* (Other).[17] My perceptions are never lived as bare concatenations of sense-data but reveal what is Other, a realm of external objects. If I were to apprehend all perceptual events simply as modifications of my body located within the perceiving organs, I would have no experience of an outer world, and thus, ultimately, even of my own body as a worldly thing. My being-in-the-world depends upon my body's self-effacing transitivity.

The From and the To

In order to shed further light upon this phenomenon I will employ an admirably simple and ontologically neutral set of terms provided by Michael Polanyi. He writes of a "from-at" or "from-to" structure, which characterizes experience in general.[18] In any act of attention we not only attend to a thematic object but from a set of cues and conditions. (Polanyi also refers to these respectively as the "explicit" and "tacit," the "focal" and "subsidiary," the "distal" and "proximal," terms of experience.) That is, in order to perceive any explicit object I must make use of means, clues, and information that are themselves unthematized and of which I may have little or no direct awareness.

For example, I recognize a soda can sitting in front of me only by virtue of utilizing, perceiving from, a vast set of perceptual particulars. I am not explicitly aware of the gradually transforming color shades that help indicate to me the three-dimensionality, materiality, and cylindrical shape of the can. I might be able to shift my attention to these bare color shades themselves, especially if I were a painter or photographer. But I would then begin to disrupt my perception of the soda can itself. I perceive the overall object insofar as the visual cues I am employing remain to a degree unthematized. To take a very different example, for you, the reader, the physical appearance of the words on this page tends to recede from focal awareness. The reader attends from these black marks to the meanings they reveal. An over attention to the shape of the letters themselves would only interfere with their function as signs. (I will analyze this phenomenon more extensively in chapter 4.)

Many of Polanyi's examples are borrowed from Gestalt psychology and refer to the subliminal use of perceptual particulars in the recognition of any object or meaning. However, this does not encompass the fullness of the "from" structure he describes. There is, as well, that body with which I perceive. As I reach out to touch the soda can in front of me there are tactile sensations and a stream of kinesthesias that course through my fingers. I am not usually aware of these as such, for they are precisely that from which I feel the hardness and solidity of the can. Normally one utilizes one's body in this subsidiary fashion, attending from it to an external world. As Polanyi writes:

> Our body is the only assembly of things known almost exclusively by relying on our awareness of them for attending to something else. . . . Every time we make sense of the world, we rely on our tacit knowledge of impacts made by the world on our body and the complex responses of our body to these impacts.[19]

It is because we experience from the body that it constitutes a nullpoint in the perceptual field.

As Polanyi recognizes in passing, elements of the "from" structure can be tacit in different ways and to different degrees.[20] The kinesthesias of my feeling hand exhibit what Polanyi calls a "marginal" presence;[21] I may be consciously aware of these sensations in an obscure fashion and could directly attend to them via a shift of focus. However, I can also utilize what Polanyi calls "subliminal" clues[22] such as the contractions of my eye muscles. While making use of such information when judging depth, these contractions are unavailable to any direct apprehension. I simply cannot bring them to explicit consciousness. Ultimately, Polanyi extends this category of the subliminal to include all neurophysiological bases of perception.[23] When gazing at a soda can I not only see from my eyes per se, but from my retinal nerves, my visual cortex. While an experimental scientist might attend to these nerve firings, they are necessarily that of which I am unaware. The from-to analysis thus exposes the fallacy involved in treating the subject as pure introspective self-presence. On the contrary, one's own grounds of experience may be more available for thematization by another.

Polanyi's terms not only illuminate the nullpoint phenomenon but the noncoincidence characteristic of reflective modes. The eye that lies at the source of the gaze experientially diverges from its mirror image. Yet this divergence is none other than that between the "from" and the "to." As that from which I perceive, my eyes play a different structural role vis-à-vis the experiential field than the reflected eyes to which I attend. Similarly, when I use my right hand to touch, it is absorbed within my structure of tacit means. Only in this way can it reveal an outer world. To say one cannot "see the seeing" or "touch the touching" is simply to recognize the noncoincidence of the "from" and the "to."

This leads to what might be termed, in analogy to physics, an "uncertainty principle" of embodiment. Just as Heisenberg recognized theoretical limitations on knowledge that could not be overcome by technical advance, such is our condition relative to lived embodiment. We simply cannot see our seeing no matter what reflective means are employed. In the case of quantum physics any attempt to measure the position and momentum of a particle necessarily changes these parameters leaving an ineluctable uncertainty. Our case bears a certain similarity; in thematizing a part of the body we necessarily change its phenomenological status. It no longer functions as part of the tacit "from" structure. But this tacit structure lies at the heart of corporeal ability. As that which operates via self-effacement, the lived body can never be a fully explicit thing.

Motility

I have derived the principle of from-to transitivity exclusively from an examination of perception. Yet in order to reconstruct the full unity of the lived body and to see whether this principle applies to it as a whole, I now take up motility and goal-directed action.

As Straus, among others, has argued extensively, the classical distinction between perception and movement is in fact highly artificial, dividing in reflection what is always united in lived experience.[24] I touch by reaching out and running my hand over the surface of an object. To see, I turn my head and let my eyes scan the landscape. Perception is itself a motor activity. Moreover, that which is perceived is always saturated by the implicit presence of motility. The spatial depth of the perceived world, the experience of objects as *there,* near or far from my body, is only possible for a being that moves through space. This is true as well of the qualitative nature of the perceived. As Straus notes, from the start we experience things about us as "alluring" or "frightening," beckoning toward us or repulsive.[25] We see chairs that offer up the prospect of rest, food that may be eaten, a cold rain that bids us stay inside.

The sensory world thus involves a constant reference to our possibilities of active response.

Given this deep interpenetration of perception and motility it should not be surprising to discover within the latter the same from-to structure that characterized the former. I will illustrate this point first in relation to a simple example: the act of taking a bite out of an apple. On reflection one can distinguish two poles of this activity: that which does the biting and that which is bitten. This is homologous to the distinction within perception between the seeing eye and the field of objects seen. And as the eye necessarily disappears from its field of endeavor, so too do the teeth while biting. That is, my teeth open up what might be termed an *actional* field. They are capable of biting not only an apple but other sorts of food, as well as fingernails, clothing, or most anything that comes within their province. But within this world revealed as thing-to-be-bitten, there is one thing I cannot thereby bite: my own teeth. My mouth cannot swallow itself, my foot kick itself, my hand grasp itself. In each case I act from these organs to the affected object or the action performed. As the very means whereby I act, these organs constitute a nullpoint within their actional field.

Admittedly, motor activity, like perception, has certain reflective possibilities. For example, one might claim that my hand can, in a sense, grasp itself, as when I clench my fist. However, self-coincidence is never total. In this case it is a question of the fingers folding back upon the palm. The hand can only achieve a full grip upon an object that spatially diverges from itself. But what of corporeal actions whose object and intent seem purely self-reflective? For example, I may clench and unclench my fist, not with the intention of gripping an external object but of building up my own hand strength. My hand seems to act upon itself. Yet there still remains a divergence between the body from and to which I act. Here noncoincidence takes a temporal rather than a spatial form. I act from my current physicality toward the ideal body, stronger and more muscular, that yet awaits me. In the structure of desire that animates action, the present condition becomes a means for achieving futural goals.

Thus, most actions manifest what I will term a *physical telos* directed away from one's own corporeal base. One acts from the here-and-now body to spatially or temporally noncoincident objects. Furthermore, this is usually accompanied by an *attentional telos* outward. One's body is rendered subsidiary, not only as a physical means to an end but within the accompanying structure of attention. As Ricoeur writes:

> Actually, when I act I am not concerned with my body. I say rather that the action "traverses" my body. . . . I am concerned less with my body

than with the product of the action: the hanged picture, the strike of the hammer on the head of a nail.[26]

My actions are motivated and organized by outer-directed concern. In order to strike the nail properly I must look at it, not my swinging hand. In deciding where the picture is to be hung I survey the walls, the colors, the spaces of my house, and contemplate the effect I am trying to achieve. My body, as the sensorimotor means of such surveying, yet recedes before this experiential primacy of ends.[27]

Admittedly, in some situations attention will shift so as to reside within the body here-and-now. For example, I may be thrust into an experience of my physical presence if, standing tiptoe on a chair, I begin to lose my balance. At once I become painfully aware of my precarious and rapidly deteriorating position. In doing my hand exercises I may find it more pleasant to forget the ideal body yet to come and simply experience my current sensations. A Zen master may follow his breathing with one-pointed attention, ignoring sensory enticements and futural goals.

Yet such experiences are not the primary ways in which most of us live out the body. They can best be understood, to use Heidegger's term, as "deficient" modes of our usual concern with the world.[28] This notion of "deficiency" has no pejorative overtones; there may be great aesthetic and contemplative benefits in attending directly to bodily activity. However, this term indicates that such modes are derivative, involving a suspension of the body's ordinary from-to telos directed away from itself. Almost from birth the infant begins to track faces and soon reach out for objects, utilizing the body as an unthematized substratum from which the world is acted upon. This transitive nature of the body is essential, inherent, a corporeal primitive. It is not something that could be secondarily added on or developed out of a field of simple presence. On the contrary, self-presencing arises from modifying this norm of transitivity.

Moreover, the self-presence we can achieve is limited, no less in action than in perception. I cannot thematize even a single movement in its entirety. Though I may concentrate on the rhythms of walking, most of the physiology of the act remains resolutely hidden from my awareness. Hume took note of this curious lacuna:

> we learn from anatomy, that the immediate object of power in voluntary motion, is not the member itself which is moved, but certain muscles, and nerves, and animal spirits, and, perhaps, something still more minute and more unknown, through which the motion is successively propagated, ere it reach the member itself whose motion is the immediate object of volition. Can there be a more certain proof, that the power, by which this whole operation is performed, so far from being directly

and fully known by an inward sentiment or consciousness, is, to the last degree, mysterious and unintelligible?[29]

I have a tacit command over my body, accomplishing without the slightest difficulty actions I could not begin to comprehend or carry out in a reflective fashion. If I attempted to walk by consciously manipulating all the proper muscles I would soon find myself incapacitated. And, taking it further, if I tried to initiate my stroll by explicitly sending out certain nerve signals from the cerebral cortex, I would not even know how to begin. All our scientific knowledge does little to change this situation. The physician still utilizes his or her body in a tacit fashion even while objectifying the body of another.[30]

Thus, in addition to its physical and attentional telos outward, action manifests what I will term a *functional telos*. In pursuing my explicit goals, I act toward the world from an unthematized functional power. As Merleau-Ponty writes, employing a Husserlian locution, "Consciousness is in the first place not a matter of 'I think that' but of 'I can.'"[31] I can walk, run, reach, grasp, speak, gesture, along with a thousand other intricate acts, though the source of these abilities remains unknown. In Merleau-Ponty's words, "The relationships between my decision and my body are, in movement, magic ones."[32] I tend to forget this magical quality precisely because it is a taken for granted base from which my actions spring.

The lived body thus constitutes a nullpoint in motor activity no less than in perceptual modes. I have described a threefold telos of motility wherein the body plays a subsidiary role. Physically, we act from a surface organ that itself is a lacuna in its actional field. In attentional terms, we ordinarily focus upon the goal of activity, not our corporeal means of accomplishment. Functionally, we rely upon a set of abilities we cannot fully thematize. Insofar as perception is itself a form of action and deeply intertwined with motility, we can retrospectively identify there the same threefold disappearance. For example, in seeing, we physically act from the eye; we attend from it to the objects of its gaze; and this vision rests upon an unknown but unproblematic "I can." Perception and motility are modulations of a singular power, the from-to structure of bodily engagement.

Ecstasis and Absence

This structure manifests itself through a broader series of variations than I will seek to trace out here in detail. For example, the body as ground of expression and communication also operates according to a from-to logic. One's gestures, facial movements, and sounds do not call for explicit thematization by self or Other—they phenomenologically recede to permit access to the message they convey (see chapter 4). Mood and emotion exhibit their own forms of transitivity. As Heidegger and Solomon indicate, moods and emotions are world-disclosive.[33] In Ricoeur's words:

> When I am moved by emotion, I do not think of my body at all. . . .
> Being afraid does not mean feeling my body shake or my heart beat; it is
> to experience the world as something to shun, as an impalpable pre-
> sence.[34]

Similarly, such corporeal states as hunger, thirst, and sexual craving are not simply "internal" twinges but modes whereby the environment stands forth. Such biological urges color the perceived world, channeling attention and activity toward potential sources of gratification. The lived body is thus first and foremost not a located thing but a path of access, a being-in-the-world. As Sartre writes, the body is "perpetually the *surpassed*."[35]

This power of transcending its own confines has formed a central theme for phenomenological authors who have labeled it with different names. Erwin Straus writes of "distance" as the "spatio-temporal form of sensing."[36] Only by projecting across a spatial and temporal distance can the sensorimotor body open up a world. Hans Jonas refers instead to a principle of "mediacy" that sentience, emotion, and motility all exhibit.[37] He cites this mediacy between subject and object, between urge and attainment, as the crucial feature that differentiates animal from vegetative life. Merleau-Ponty, influenced by Husserl, refers to a "basic" or "operative" intentionality founded in the body and prior to explicit judgments.[38]

Yet the notion of intentionality brings with it unnecessary philosophical baggage. It was predicated by Brentano as precisely that trait which distinguished mentality from the physical[39] and has at times implied reference to an inexistent object immanent within the subject's mind. Such connotations are directly opposed to the corporeal world-relatedness I have been exploring. While free of such resonances, terms such as "distance" and "mediacy," seemingly mundane and unproblematic, fail to highlight the radical paradox of the present-absent body. In their place, I will choose a term derived from the Greek, and more recently employed by Heidegger: *ecstasis.* This word includes within it the root *ek,* meaning "out," and *stasis,* meaning "to stand." The ecstatic is that which stands out. This admirably describes the operation of the lived body. The body always has a determinate stance—it is that whereby we are located and defined. But the very nature of the body is to project outward from its place of standing. From the "here" arises a perceptual world of near and far distances. From the "now" we inhabit a meaningful past and a futural realm of projects and goals.[40]

In this ecstatic nature of corporeality can be discovered the first reason that the body is forgotten in experience. Heidegger writes, "There are coverings-up which are accidental; there are also some which are necessary, grounded in what the thing discovered consists in."[41] I have been discussing the latter sort of covering-up. The body conceals itself precisely in the act of revealing what is Other. The very presencing of the world and of the body as an object within it is always correlative with this primordial absence.

In exploring this intertwining of presence and absence, etymology can again play a suggestive role. The word *absence* comes from the Latin *esse,* or "being," and *ab,* meaning "away." An absence is the being-away of something. The lived body, as ecstatic in nature, is that which is away from itself. Yet this absence is not equivalent to a simple void, a mere lack of being. The notion of being is after all present in the very word *absence.* The body could not be away, stand outside, unless it had a being and stance to begin with. It is thus never fully eradicated from the experiential world. Otherwise I would not even know I had a body.

In this context, my employment of the Husserlian metaphor of the nullpoint was provisional and potentially misleading. The body is not a sheer nullity either within the field of action or awareness. To clarify this point I will pause briefly to summarize the modes of presence one's own body retains. This will enable me both to criticize and supplement the notion of the nullpoint and to arrive at a more complex model of embodiment.

Presencings

I have already touched on several ways in which the body, even when unthematized, remains indirectly or marginally available to experience. Though it may be nowhere manifest within the perceptual field, my body is indicated as the orientational center in relation to which everything else takes its place. As a result, I come away with as precise a reading of my own location within the environment as I do for any appearing object. I experience myself as always situated *here,* not spread throughout existence like a god or pure mind. Precisely insofar as the corporeal nullpoint is like a point it could not be a total nullity; a point is that which has definite location.

The body is also defined through its actional fields. The use-qualities

and accessibility of surrounding objects always refer back to my corporeal powers. To see something as reachable and thereby open to my
use is to implicitly experience my body's capacity of reach. If I become
weakened or paralyzed, the quality of the world is equivalently transformed; objects now recede, mock me, proclaim my inability.

Nor is all reference to the body indirect, routed through an external
world. My body is always a field of immediately lived sensation,
Empfindnisse, to use Husserl's term.[42] Its presence is fleshed out by a
ceaseless stream of kinesthesias, cutaneous and visceral sensations, defining my body's space and extension and yielding information about
position, balance, state of tension, desire, and mood. Oliver Sacks describes the case of a woman with a rare form of polyneuritis who had
lost the proprioceptive sense of her body.[43] While she was capable of
employing visual, auditory, and vestibular cues, the internal feel of embodiment was missing. She experienced her body as dead, derealized,
not her own, looked for her arm in one place and was surprised to find it
elsewhere. In her words, "I feel my body is blind and deaf to itself . . . it
has no sense of itself."[44] This experience of loss illuminates, by way of
contrast, the subtle coenesthetic presence the body maintains even when
ecstatically caught up in the world. Moreover, such coenesthesias can be
explicitly thematized either through choice or involuntary changes. As I
will discuss in chapter 3, situations of extreme pain, fatigue, or other
organic disturbances especially draw attention to our bodily states.

In addition to this coenesthetic awareness, we have access to multiple
modes of self-observation mediated by outer-directed senses. I can employ the reflective surfaces of the world: mirrors, bodies of water,
photographs, etc. The gaze of another also initiates self-reflection. I apprehend myself as embodied and defined when I look into the eyes of
another looking at me (see chapter 3). And, as Merleau-Ponty points
out, such intersubjectivity draws upon an intersubjectivity implicit
within my own body.[45] In gazing upon or touching itself, my body actualizes "a sort of reflection."[46] Though there is no absolute coincidence
between the observing and observed body, there is no absolute division
either. These are dimensions of a single lived body.

This folding back of the body upon itself is only possible because the
body is an extended structure containing within it a multiplicity of parts
and powers. Thus, my sensorimotor capabilities can reflect one upon
another; my eyes can look down upon my hands, my hands can touch
each other or reach up to touch my eyes. If the body were simply a point
source, an eye at the moment of sight or a fingertip at the moment of
touching, I could not gain this perspective on self.

Hence, the metaphor of the body as nullpoint requires dual supplementation; it is never a pure nullity in experience, but neither is it simply a point. Every moment invokes the synthetic operation of a highly diverse range of functions. This ineradicable presence of the body-as-a-whole has to some degree been covered over by my previous examples, which have largely focused on individual organs. To achieve a fuller understanding of bodily presence-absence it is necessary to broaden the context of my discussion. From the body considered as originary point, I will introduce the notion of the corporeal field.

The Corporeal Field

As Richard Zaner points out (referring to the work of Kurt Goldstein), the use of any organ necessarily involves the enlistment of the rest of the body in a "background attitude."[47] When I gaze at a landscape I dwell most fully in my eyes. Yet this is only possible because my back muscles hold my spine erect, my neck muscles adjust my head into the proper position for viewing. My feet, my legs, my arms, all lend their support. My other perceptual senses flesh out the scene I witness with sound and warmth, even if my attention is centered on visual characteristics. My whole body provides the background that supports and enables the point of corporeal focus. As such, the body itself is not a point but an organized field in which certain organs and abilities come to prominence while others recede.[48]

We can thus employ the notion of the figure-ground gestalt to characterize not only the body's field of experience but the structure of the experiencing body itself. The figure-ground relations inherent in the body are typified by a high degree of complexity. Within any given corporeal gestalt there may be, and often is, more than one prominent focus *from* which we act. For example, in driving a car I am constantly relying upon my gaze. At the same time, my arms and hands steer the wheel in immediate, unreflective response to the road. My feet play across the accelerator and brake, modulating my speed appropriately. My very life depends on this prethematic synthesis of eyes, hands, feet, a series of linked corporeal foci.

In addition, at any given time the bodily field is capable of embracing more than one actional gestalt. For example, while driving I may turn on the radio and soon find myself singing along. My ears and mouth here act as the linked foci of a corporeal gestalt elicited by the music. This second structure does not interfere with that involved in driving because of a certain intergestalt fit. While focal in relation to the music, the ears and mouth are relegated to an inessential role in driving. Conversely, the eyes, hands, and feet so central to driving play a background role relative to listening to music. This complementarity of figure-ground demands allows the two gestalts to coexist harmoniously. (This would not be the case if I tried, for example, to watch television while driving: competing focal demands would be placed on one set of eyes, causing disruption of one or both activities.) While maintaining their independence, coexisting gestalts may yet interpenetrate through pre-reflective corporeal syntheses. I may find myself accelerating when a fast song comes on the radio; the very temporality and spatiality of the road are altered by different sorts of music.

Thus, at any given time the body manifests a gestalt structure. But within the gestalt of a single activity there may be several corporeal foci drawn together. Furthermore, the general corporeal field may include several perceptual or actional gestalts coexisting and exerting mutual pulls. As has been suggested, this complex field structure allows for more modes of corporeal self-presencing than if the body were simply a point, a nullpoint. The diverse powers available to me allow me to re-flect back upon my body from a multitude of discrete perspectives. However, this field structure also allows for a more complex pattern of absence than previously analyzed. To explain, I will return to the main theme of this chapter: the self-effacement of the surface body.

Forms of Disappearance

My discussion of the body's figure-ground relations implies the exist-ence of at least two complementary forms of absence: not only that ad-hering to the body's focal organs but that characterizing the background of the corporeal field. To illustrate, I will go back to the example with which this chapter began. I noted that when looking across an open space toward a tree in the distance, my eyes nowhere appeared within my visual field. I went on to explore that one fact in depth. But that hardly constitutes a full description of the self-effacement operative in that moment. In such a situation I would likely be relatively unaware not only of my eyes but of my legs and feet, the back muscles supporting me, my torso at large. Unused sensory capacities such as taste would similar-ly recede from apprehension. These corporeal regions and powers are forgotten not because they are focal points from which I act and experi-ence but because at this moment they are precisely *not* bodily foci. Dwelling within the power of sight as my primary mode of world-dis-closure, I relegate much of my body to the status of neutral background. This corporeal background, even more than the background of a per-ceptual field, tends to disappear from explicit awareness.

The corporeal background is itself a highly complex phenomenon composed of different functional elements. Certain aspects of the background will operate to provide crucial support for bodily foci of action or perception. The muscle groups that support the head, enabling vision, are an example of this. Elements of the corporeal background can also be utilized in activity irrelevant to the attentional center. I may, for example, keep tying knots in a piece of string while concentrating on the visual spectacle. Though it constitutes a second actional focus, this knot-tying gestalt remains a background in terms of the overall field of attention.

In other cases organs and powers are simply put out of play so as not to interfere with the primary locus of engagement. To take a better look at the tree I may have stopped walking and ceased a distracting conversation with my companion. My mouth and legs fall still, permitting attention to flood out through my eyes. For me to engage in any activity there are a countless number of other actions I must cease, skills and motor schemas I leave unused, corporeal regions I render quiescent. Those regions and actions nonetheless remain a part of my corporeal background understood in the broad sense. They belong to my bodily "I can," available for use at the appropriate moment.

Having characterized the corporeal background, I can now identify the two complementary forms of self-concealment that mark the surface body. One I will call *focal disappearance*. This refers to the self-effacement of bodily organs when they form the focal origin of a perceptual or actional field. An example is the invisibility of the eye within the visual field it generates. I have spent the bulk of the chapter describing modes of focal disappearance and their "from-to" or "ecstatic" structure. In contrast, I have recently been discussing what I will now term *background disappearance*. Bodily regions can disappear because they are *not* the focal origin of our sensorimotor engagements but are backgrounded in the corporeal gestalt: that is, they are for the moment relegated to a supportive role, involved in irrelevant movement, or simply put out of play.

I here employ the term *disappearance* rather than *absence,* for I have given the latter a more general significance. *Absence,* according to its etymology, refers to all the ways in which the body can *be away* from itself. One manner is simply through disappearing from self-awareness. Disappearance is thus a form of absence. It is not, however, the only form. As I will discuss in chapter 3, certain modes of experiential appearance are marked by paradoxical self-opposition, and hence their own sort of being-away or "absence."

In addition, my technical use of the term *disappearance* should be distinguished from its ordinary sense. Customarily, *disappearance* implies the vanishing of something that was originally present to the gaze. This is not the case with the phenomena I am discussing. For example, it is not a matter of the eye once having appeared in its visual field, only subsequently to vanish—it is simply that which never shows itself for structural reasons. *Disappearance,* in my usage, trades on the frequent use of *dis-* as a straightforward prefix of negation. To "disappear" in this sense is simply to not-appear.

My characterization of the two modes of disappearance should not obscure the important experiential dissimilarities between them. Just as there are different forms of presencing, so things can absence in very different ways. To use an example adapted from J. H. van den Berg, as I climb a mountainside, straining, searching for my footing, my legs and feet manifest a focal disappearance.[49] I do not attend to them, but from them, feeling for the slippery rocks, seeking a toehold. My consciousness spreads out from my lower extremities, and they disappear in this ecstatic movement. This is quite different from when I sit quietly reading, my legs lying still. My legs are then enveloped in a background disappearance; awareness is simply withdrawn from their situation. Or there is my previous example of gazing toward a tree, eyes in focal disappearance. If I were to shut my eyes to better hear the sounds of nature, sight would now enter a background mode. In the former case my eyes disappear in the act of lighting up the world. But in the latter case they disappear into darkness; I have abandoned their disclosive abilities.

The Complemental Series

The structural relationship between these two modes of disappearance can be described by employing a concept used by Freud, the *complemental series*. In examining the origin of neurosis, Freud refused to choose between constitutional or experiential factors as the exclusive etiological mode. He writes:

> As regards their causation, instances of neurotic illness fall into a series within which the two factors . . . are represented in such a manner that if there is more of the one there is less of the other."[50]

Certain patients, lacking any clear constitutional predisposition, fall ill as a result of a strongly detrimental environment. At the other end of the spectrum, Freud asserts that neurosis can arise in patients with an inherent developmental tendency in this direction "however carefully their lives had been sheltered."[51] In addition, there are less clear-cut instances that show differing degrees of both factors in operation. A complemental series, as described by Freud, exhibits a full range of intermediate examples, as well as those of the polar extremes. Yet there is a certain summative constancy at work. In all cases, "the diminishing intensity of one factor is balanced by an increasing intensity of the other."[52] In producing neurosis, for example, a lesser constitutional predisposition must have been counteracted by an increase in environmental stressors. A complemental series is characterized by the origin of a certain result through the balanced operation of two different causal factors.

The phenomenon under discussion fits well the model of a complemental series. A certain result, the disappearance of the surface body from thematic awareness, arises from the operation of two different etiological factors: focal and background disappearance. Moreover, these two factors stand in an inverse relationship whose necessity surpasses that of Freud's example. That is, a strongly detrimental environment in no way assures that the neurotic does not also have a powerful constitutional predisposition at play. The increase of one factor is not structurally and necessarily linked to the decrease of the other. However, in the example I gave it is. Insofar as a part of my body is taken up focally, it can no longer play a background role relative to that activity, and vice versa.[53] As I close my eyes, their absorption into a background disappearance entails their simultaneous removal from focal operation. In my ongoing use of the notion of the complemental series, I will thus slightly modify Freud's original formulation. I define a *complemental series* as the emergence of a phenomenon from the balanced operation of two etiological factors, wherein the rising of one is necessarily correlative with the other's decline.

In relation to the body surface taken as a whole, not just a specific organ, both etiological factors will always play a role. As a functional gestalt, the body maintains an ongoing figure-ground structure and will thus exhibit both forms of disappearance. It is possible, though, to recognize certain sorts of activities in which one or the other mode predominates. For example, when taking an early morning walk in the forest I am caught up in the sounds and smells of this world. Striding vigorously down the trail, I pause to pick wildflowers and dip my hand into a nearby brook. It is as if I dwelled fully within my corporeality, existing its sensory powers and reawakening its muscles. My body is taken up primarily in its focal disappearance as a variegated mode of disclosing the world. This would be particularly refreshing if the previous week had been spent at the typewriter. There, thoughts and fingers alone in motion, I ignore all sensory allurements that might distract me. I perch in a chair for hours suspending large portions of my corporeal existence in order to proceed with my specific task. This body is largely placed into background disappearance though I still use limited regions and maintain a marginal awareness of the potentials from which I hold back. Such activities, respectively emphasizing focal or background disappearance, define the extremes of a complemental series filled with intermediate cases.

In addition to characterizing different forms of activity, these modes of disappearance can be used to distinguish between various bodily regions. Different parts of the body will tend to recede in different ways, defining a complementary series in anatomico-functional terms. I have hitherto concentrated largely on key organs of the body like the eyes and the hands. Exhibiting highly complex sensorimotor capabilities, these organs often play a focal role in perceiving and acting. They thus lend themselves to a focal disappearance. This is true in general of my face, which serves as an originary locus of communication and perception. In contrast, my torso, legs, and feet are often enveloped in a background disappearance. So too is the backside of the body, given the forward-directedness of our sensorimotor organs. As Charles Sherrington points out in his classic of neurophysiology, *The Integrative Action of the Nervous System,* animals whose bodies are organized along a single axis tend to manifest a "leading segment."[54] The appendages are adapted for locomotion in this direction, and the sense receptors of this leading segment develop to a remarkable degree. The animal is thus able to react sensitively to what is approaching, in advance of immediate physical encounter. In this focus upon that which lies spatially and temporally ahead, the back of the body is comparatively forgotten. It is absorbed in background disappearance.

Admittedly, there will be large individual and cultural variations in this scheme. Different people will utilize their physique in divergent ways, perhaps accentuating regions that others overlook. Entire societies also differ greatly from one another in their appropriation of the body. There are, for example, cultures that make much more extensive use of the sense of smell or hearing than we do in our visually-oriented society. Cultures even differ on the bodily seat of consciousness or soul. Most modern Westerners would experience this unequivocally as the head. But the Greeks found this center within the chest, and the Zen meditator develops the *hara,* located within the belly, as the wellspring of enlightened experience and action.[55]

Yet these variations are possible only within, and are limited by, the common structure of the human body. Its sensory organs, its forward-directedness, its muscular capacities, are prearticulations upon which all cultures must build. As such, one can trace out a "phenomenological anatomy" of the lived body, characterizing its different regions according to their usual forms of presence and absence and the modes of world-relation they permit or encourage. My distinction between organs that naturally lend themselves to a focal versus a background disappearance is but the crude beginning of such a mapping.[56] Nor is this anything like a complete survey of corporeal absence, the subject to which I restrict myself in this work. For example, I have dealt so far only with the disappearances adhering to the bodily surface. There are, as well, disappearances characteristic of the inner body. As I will discuss in chapter 2, visceral organs manifest their own pattern of withdrawal from personal awareness and control.

Incorporation

Before turning attention toward these corporeal depths, my model of the surface body requires a further supplementation. In commencing a phenomenological anatomy, I have moved from the simple to the progressively more complex. Beginning with the perceptual taken in isolation, I have introduced the body as seat of motility and praxis. The model of embodiment as nullpoint, based on the functioning of individual organs, has given way to a recognition of the corporeal field. Nonetheless, the body I have so far portrayed remains largely a static one. That is, I have operated as if the body were composed of a fixed mass of organs and abilities, only shifting its patterns of use to foreground or background a particular region. But in fact, the body as a whole is always shifting. As Leibniz writes, "all bodies are in a state of perpetual flux like rivers, and the parts are continually entering in and passing out."[57] This flux of parts can be understood not only in a physical but a phenomenological sense. The lived body constantly transforms its sensorimotor repertoire by acquiring novel skills and habits. In its use of tools and machines the body supplements itself through annexing artificial organs. A phenomenological anatomy cannot then be thought of as fixed over time, or even confined by the physical boundaries of the flesh. It must take account of the body as living process.

Skills

Once again, the concept of disappearance provides a key for understanding these corporeal transformations. To illustrate this point I will begin by examining the acquisition of a skill. The initial stages of mastering a new skill usually involve a complex series of thematizations. If, for example, I am learning to swim, I pay explicit attention to certain rules of performance. I am told to cup my hands, lift my arms from the water, and breathe to one side. Moreover, I attend to the examples provided by others. As Ryle[58] and Polanyi[59] have pointed out, to "know how" to do something need not imply that one intellectually understands or can explain all that one does. Watching others swim may teach me more than their words. Finally, even this watching must give way before the body's need for direct performance. I imitate the swimmer's gestures and at last, with misgivings, take the plunge myself. As I try to swim I consciously monitor my own movements, making sure I am kicking and breathing correctly. The problematic nature of these novel gestures tends to provoke explicit body awareness (see chapter 3).

Yet the successful acquisition of a new ability coincides with a phenomenological effacement of all this. The thematization of rules, of examples, of my own embodiment, falls away once I truly know how to swim. I no longer need think about cupping my hands or the right style of breathing. This now comes without conscious effort, allowing my focus to be directed elsewhere.

Such a process of progressive experiential disappearance characterizes the acquisition of higher cognitive skills, not merely those of an immediate physical nature. For example, the learning of a new language involves its own structure of copious thematization. I study rules of grammar, memorize the conjugation of verbs, pore over lists of vocabulary words. I learn where to move my tongue to pronounce the proper sounds; my body is again rendered perspicuous by difficulty.

Yet, as with swimming, when the language is truly learned, all this apparatus can fall away. I find myself actually reading a book with comprehension. I can attend to the story line itself rather than my own halting efforts at translation. Where before the words were opaque, their foreign look and sound consciously thematized, I now experience *to* the meaning they disclose (see chapter 4).

This skill acquisition is accomplished via a process I will term *incorporation.* From the Latin *corpus,* or "body," the etymology of this word literally means to "bring within a body." A skill is finally and fully learned when something that once was extrinsic, grasped only through explicit rules or examples, now comes to pervade my own corporeality. My arms know how to swim, my mouth can at last speak the language. This embodied aspect is already suggested by the etymological root of the word *language* in the word for *tongue*—when I finally master a foreign language, it is as if all the instruction, study, and practice finally have sunk right into my tongue. A skill has been incorporated into my bodily "I can."

If absence lies at the heart of the lived body, then any extension of its sensorimotor powers must necessarily involve an extension of absence. This then explains the experiential disappearance that accompanies the incorporation of skills. The unproblematic use of a skill coincides with its participation in the body's focal disappearance. Whereas in the stage of learning I act *to* the skill qua thematized goal, in mastery it becomes that *from* which I operate upon the world. I experience from my command of a new language to the works of literature it allows me to read. Having learned to swim, it is now the taken-for-granted means whereby I head out for the other side of the lake.

Moreover, when not actively in use, an acquired skill participates in background disappearance. It recedes as a part of my bodily repertoire temporarily put out of play while I employ different schemas. Thus, on a cold day I "background" the possibility of swimming. Like other structures in background disappearance the mastered skill yet remains a part of the "I can," exerting its subliminal field of force. The lake outside my window still looks different than in my preswimming days, when it could not be crossed and offered no access.

These bodily transformations are not accomplished via an intellectual "flash of understanding"[60] but through something akin to a sedimentary process. Over time, that which is acted out, rehearsed, and repeated seeps into one's organismic ground. As Ricoeur points out, this sedimentation could never take place by a sheer act of will. The will "can only activate or hinder a specific formative function which we might well call involuntary: *practice* is what has this 'spontaneous' power."[61]

Incorporation thus has a temporal significance. The body masters a novel skill by incorporating its own corporeal history of hours and days spent in practice. I act from not just my present organs, but a bodily past that tacitly structures my responses.[62] As Ricoeur writes, "What once was analyzed, thought, and willed drifts bit by bit into the realm of that which I have never known or willed."[63] In Polanyi's terms, the "to" over time can become the "from." This process of temporal self-incorporation can give rise both to novelty and stasis. As discussed, incorporation is the very means whereby new abilities are acquired, unlocking novel aspects of the world. However, it is also via incorporation that abilities sediment into fixed habits. As a result of ongoing patterns of action, the body can develop automatic tendencies to repeat. I may fall into unreflective habits concerning waking up and going to sleep, conducting myself on the job, interacting with colleagues, exercising, or relaxing. The vast reach of the "I can" contracts into the "I do," that region of body possibility I actually use. Nor, because of the nature of incorporation, is it easy to excise or even recognize such habits. Over time they simply disappear from view. They are enveloped within the structure of the taken-for-granted body from which I in*habit* the world.

Technologies

Incorporation manifests not only a temporal but a spatial reach. The body is capable of incorporating within its phenomenological domain objects that remain spatially discrete. This is evidenced by the example of the tool, whose existential significance was emphasized by Heidegger.[64] The tool, he writes, is something "ready-to-hand" (*zuhanden*), part of an equipmental structure that tends to withdraw from our explicit attention. We concern ourselves primarily with the work or product "towards-which" we labor.

Though Heidegger does not explicitly refer to the body in this famous discussion, his terminology is highly suggestive. This notion of the "ready-to-hand" refers us implicitly back to the hand itself. As we have seen, one's own hands, as the means with which one works upon the world, themselves withdraw from explicit thematization. The disappearance of the hand-held tool is none other than an offshoot of bodily disappearance closing over the incorporated instrument.

This is illustrated by the example of the blind man's stick, referred to by Polanyi[65] and Merleau-Ponty.[66] When first employing such a stick one experiences *to* it as an external object exerting impacts upon the hand. Yet as the tool is mastered one begins to feel through it to the experiential field it discloses.[67] As Merleau-Ponty writes:

> The blind man's stick has ceased to be an object for him, and is no longer perceived for itself; its point has become an area of sensitivity, extending the scope and active radius of touch, and providing a parallel to sight.[68]

The stick thus enters into focal disappearance, becoming part of the "from" structure of the body.[69] This occurs as well with more complex instruments; for example, I do not attend to the telephone but to the person with whom it enables me to speak. My natural organs are modified and supplemented via the incorporation of such artificial extensions. This internal relation of bodily organ and tool is suggested by the Greek usage of one word, *organon,* to refer to both.[70]* Nor is this relation severed when I abandon an instrument, for example, laying down the telephone receiver. The apparatus yet retains the marginal presence characteristic of background disappearance. That is, while momentarily put out of play, instrumental capabilities, no less than the skills indigenous to my body, remain a part of my corporeal "I can." I can speak with my friend across the country through the amplified voice and hearing the telephone provides. Even if I choose to background this possibility, refusing to call for long stretches of time, there is yet a significance to my very holding back. Our relationship unfolds in the space created by our technologically supplemented bodies, not merely that of our natural flesh.[71]* [Note: an asterisk is used to mark footnotes which take up significant issues not treated within the main body of the text.]

The term "incorporation" seems to imply an absorptive process operating in a unilateral direction. Via a phenomenological osmosis, the body brings within itself novel abilities, its own temporal history, and tools that remain spatially discrete. However, incorporation is the result of a rich dialectic wherein the world transforms my body, even as my body transforms its world. Why did I first learn to swim? Because the lake outside my window invited me to do so. I acquired a new language because it was called for by the appearance of books I had to read. The demands and solicitations of the world gradually lead me to reshape the ability-structure of my body.

This is true as well in the case of technologies. We build machines because the resistance of the world demands a supplementing of our physical powers. For example, the sheer distances we encounter, incommensurate with the structure of our legs, call forth our technologies of transportation and communication. This dialectical body-world relation is concretized even in the simplest of instruments. Ordinarily, any tool will have one end specifically adapted to our human anatomy; the handle of a saw is designed to fit the hand. However, the other end is adapted to the world upon which we act. The sawteeth must "fit" the wood if they are to cut properly. The line, sinker, and bait must fit the fish. To incorporate a tool is to redesign one's extended body until its extremities expressly mesh with the world.[72]*

Thus, the from-to movement of the ecstatic body opens us to reciprocal exchange. I go from my tacit embodiment to a thematically present world. However, the world I discover leads me to redesign the body itself. Just as the "from" incorporates what once was "to," the "to" rebounds to transform the "from."

Given this fluidity of body-world relations, the disappearances discussed in these pages constantly overrun the limits of our flesh. As Elaine Scarry points out, the very house in which one dwells is both a reconstruction of the surrounding world to fit the body and an enlargement of our own physical structure.[73] Its walls form a second protective skin, windows acting as artificial senses, entire rooms, like the bedroom or kitchen, devoted to a single bodily function. As such, the experience of one's own house will be marked by corporeal effacement. As I gaze through the windows they are in focal disappearance, the means from which I look upon the world. The bedroom, forgotten during the busy afternoon, recedes into a sort of background disappearance.

As I go through the day, my extended body ebbs and flows, now absorbing things, now casting them back onto shore. I do not notice my body, but neither do I, for the most part, notice the bed on which I sleep, the clothes I wear, the chair on which I sit down to breakfast, the car I drive to work. I live in bodies beyond bodies, clothes, furniture, room, house, city, recapitulating in ever expanding circles aspects of my corporeality. As such, it is not simply my surface organs that disappear but entire regions of the world with which I dwell in intimacy.

2

The Recessive Body

Life, which seeks its own continuance, tends to repair itself without our help. It mends its spiders' webs when they have been torn; it reestablishes in us the conditions of health, and itself heals the injuries inflicted upon it. . . . The essential, maternal basis of our conscious life is therefore that unconscious life which we perceive no more than the outer hemisphere of the moon perceives the earth, while all the time indissolubly and eternally bound to it.

H. F. Amiel, *Journal,* August 9, 1862

I have hitherto dwelled upon the surface, the outside of the body. Our powers of perception, motility, and expression project from a physical surface laid open to the world. Through technologies this surface extends even beyond the skin, annexing artificial organs.

I now turn attention to our corporeal depths. With the word *depth* I signify both a physical locale and a phenomenological style. In physical terms, my body surface envelops a hidden mass of internal organs and processes. The visceral functions that unfold in these bodily depths are crucial for sustaining my life. Yet such processes constitute a hidden depth vis-à-vis myself as experiencer. They are largely unavailable to my conscious awareness and command. In the depths of sleep, in the depths of my prenatal past, I am given over wholly to this unconscious vitality. Any examination of corporeal disappearance must take such phenomena into account.

Yet, such phenomena have been neglected in many treatments of the lived body. The most influential writer on embodiment, Merleau-Ponty, is a case in point. He treats the person as essentially embodied, not a pure consciousness contingently encased. Yet the lived body he describes is never complete. There is little discussion of metabolism, sleep, visceral processes, birth, and death. As the title of his central work indicates, Merleau-Ponty is most interested in the phenomenology of perception and the functions of motility and expression with which it intertwines. He is thereby able to show how traditional epistemological and existential themes are enriched by an analysis of corporeal being. Yet, by virtue of this emphasis on the "higher" and ecstatic regions of the body, the Merleau-Pontian subject still bears a distant resemblance to its Cartesian predecessor, never fully fleshed out with bone and guts.[1] (I will discuss this point at greater length toward the end of the chapter.)

Ecstatic functions such as perception will necessarily stand out for the phenomenological observer. For such functions are most prominent in shaping the experiential field. The power of the gaze, for example, structures much of my experience of spatiality, objects, and other people and in turn is visible to others as a core of my subjectivity. The same cannot be said of my spleen. This organ gives rise to no projective field. Moreover, it is largely unavailable to my own awareness or that of others. Hence it may easily be overlooked within a phenomenology of experience, even one in which the experiencer is existentialized and re-embodied.

Yet the work of a Merleau-Ponty also sets the stage for the remedy of this neglect. The move to the lived body breaks the spell that consciousness has woven over post-Cartesian and post-Kantian philosophy. Insofar as I am an embodied being, I am caught up in a prethetic, ambiguous, and practical involvement with the world. My self-presencing in consciousness will thus be lined by a multiplicity of absences: the unseen sides of the perceiver and perceived, the unknown motivators of my action, the indefinite horizons of praxical engagement. Reflective awareness rests on that which necessarily eludes it. The phenomenologist of the body is already, and necessarily, a hermeneut. To explore the region of the body most hidden from awareness is merely to extend this hermeneutical approach.

To focus my discussions of this inner body, I will concentrate upon a paradigmatic though rather unglamorous function: digestion. In order to avoid false generalizations, this example will be supplemented from time to time with references to other organ systems. The category of the "visceral" understood broadly includes not only the organs of the digestive system but of the respiratory, cardiovascular, urogenital, and endocrine systems, along with the spleen. But to examine every system with its different ways of withdrawing or surfacing to consciousness, its modes of escaping or complying with personal will, would constitute a large project in itself. (Buytendijk's *Prolegomena to an Anthropological Physiology*[2] represents a start in this direction.) Remaining with my central theme, I will attempt to elucidate a mode of bodily disappearance, not to trace out a comprehensive phenomenology. On the other hand, because of the relative paucity of literature dealing with this topic, I will engage in a more detailed phenomenology of the inner organs than was necessary in regard to surface functions.

As in chapter 1, I will first examine the perceptual characteristics of this corporeal region, then its motor form. Rather than obscuring the deep unity of experience and action this method will only confirm it. It will emerge, as was noted in relation to the ecstatic body, that visceral perception and motility share a common structure. Once uncovered, this structure will be defined, expanded via further examples, and situated philosophically.

Digestion: A Phenomenological Example

In the first chapter I briefly used the example of a person eating an apple. At that time the analysis was confined to a particular climactic and transitory point in this process: the act of biting. I will now widen the horizons of this act, permitting it to expand backward and forward in time and subjecting it to a deeper scrutiny:

After a few hours of work my thoughts begin to wander. There is a slight gnawing in my stomach, a longing, seemingly emanating from the mouth, for something to eat. My limbs are growing heavy, my mind a bit dull. I am only dimly aware of all this but soon find myself arising from my seat, heading in the direction of the cafeteria.

Arriving there, my gaze fastens on a particularly appetizing apple. I sit down, cut it in sections with my pocket knife, and take a bite. I revel in its sweetness for a moment, but soon I am lost in the newspaper I brought with me. I absentmindedly chew and swallow . . .

Let us stop for a moment the sensorimotor flow. What has occurred so far can be assimilated into the paradigm previously developed of the ecstatic, incorporative body. Though I may have briefly thematized my hunger sensations or consequent movements, for the most part I lived from them to the objects of pursuit: the cafeteria, the apple. Corporeal regions thus entered a focal disappearance as the origin of perceptions and actions directed toward the world. Other body regions, used only supportively or put out of play, receded into background disappearance. I forgot my legs as I sat down. Even the eating became an attentional background when I shifted awareness to the newspaper. External objects were incorporated into these modes of absence; the knife became a part of my tacit embodiment when I used it to cut.

However, such modes of disappearance hardly exhaust the absences that haunt my body. One is tempted to regard the gustatory example as completed at the moment of swallowing only because this moment inaugurates an even deeper absence . . .

I have a slight sense of the apple piece sliding down the back of my throat. Past a certain point this fades away. That bit is simply gone. My attention is already on the newspaper and the next bite of apple. I finish eating. After a few minutes, I burp and feel a bit of acid burning in my throat. There is (as it was a big apple), a sense of fullness in the midsection along with a renewed energy flooding through my limbs. Imperceptibly over the next hour, and as if of its own accord, the sensation of fullness disappears, leaving my middle in a vague neutrality. Some time later this is punctuated by a mild crampy sensation that pulls my attention downward. I think, though I am not at all sure, that this may be associated with the apple I ate. Perhaps it didn't agree with me.

Throughout most of this time my awareness of the digestive process has been virtually nonexistent. I am involved in my thoughts and outer-directed projects. Yet many hours after eating, I gradually become aware of a new project: the need to find a bathroom. There is a sense of increasing heaviness and fullness near my rectum calling for action. For the moment I suppress the urge as I am busy at work. At first this is easy, and the sensation temporarily subsides. However, over time the demand strengthens, and finding a nearby facility I allow what remains of the apple, and all else I ate, to reemerge in its mysteriously transformed state.

Visceral Perception

According to a scheme employed in physiology, the body's sensory powers can be divided into three categories. *Interoception* refers to all sensations of the viscera, that is, the internal organs of the body.[3] It is usually distinguished both from *exteroception*, our five senses open to the external world, and *proprioception*, our sense of balance, position, and muscular tension, provided by receptors in muscles, joints, tendons, and the inner ear. In this section I will describe three essential features that structure the interoceptive field; I will term these features respectively *qualitative reduction, spatial ambiguity,* and *spatiotemporal discontinuity.*

Qualitative Reduction

Ordinarily that which enters the interoceptive field is simultaneously lost to the exteroceptive. Before swallowing the apple I can see, touch, smell, and taste it in all its crimson-tart vividness. Once swallowed, these possibilities are swallowed up as well. I can occasionally, and perhaps unpleasantly, hear or smell evidence of my digestive activity. As in the above example, I can even catch a taste via esophageal reflux. Yet aside from such intermittent and muted evidences, the incorporation of an object into the visceral space involves its withdrawal from exteroceptive experience.

The perceptual field into which the object is received is limited compared to that of the surface body. Interoception does not share the multidimensionality of exteroception. The latter utilizes five sense-modalities which, though tightly interwoven in everyday praxis, have radically divergent spatiotemporal and qualitative properties. Interoception is not devoid of an expressive range and utilizes, physiologists tell us, a variety of sense-receptor types, including mechanoreceptors, nociceptors, and even some thermoreceptors. Yet these are experienced as modulating a single dimension of perception, i.e., "inner sensation," rather than opening onto distinct perceptual worlds.

Furthermore, the qualitative range of this dimension is reduced even when compared to any single exteroceptive mode. Touch, the most analogous form of surface perception, includes within it a huge variety of sensory statements. My acutely articulate skin yields a panoply of tickles, itches, pains, sensations of light and deep pressure, warmth and cold, slow and fast vibrations. The interoceptive vocabulary is not as well developed. In the above example, the stomach and intestines yield a feeling of fullness and cramping. The esophagus burns with an acid reflux. Yet this comes close to exhausting the ordinary sensory experiences of this region. In physiological terms, the viscera have a greatly decreased number and variety of sensory receptors compared to the surface body, as well as a limited repertoire of motor responses. Experientially, one notices a certain crudeness and generality to most of the messages received. This is a common problem for diagnosing physicians. An experience of "tightness" in the chest could signal any of a number of cardiac, respiratory, muscular, or even alimentary difficulties, given the imprecision of interoception.

The limited interoceptive vocabulary largely centers around sensations that are affectively charged. Through my outer-directed senses I can survey the exteroceptive field without immediate emotional response. The separation between the perceiver and the perceived makes possible a dispassionate scan. By contrast, visceral sensations grip me from within, often exerting an emotional insistence. As the example suggests, it is the discomforting or painful sensations that speak up most clearly: the crampy stomach, the heartburn, the insistent need for defecation. Like the infant who cries in displeasure but lapses into contentment silently, the viscera seem most able and most articulate in relation to dysfunction (see chapter 3 below). The biological/existential significance of this is clear. It is at times of dysfunction that an insistent and aversive call is needed to compel reparatory action.

While my interoceptive vocabulary is thus most developed in relation to pain, it is limited even here when compared to the body surface. My skin is susceptible to the most exquisite and differentiated tortures if it is cut, burned, pricked, tickled, stretched, struck, pinched. The inner organs exhibit comparatively restricted modes of discomfort. A particular viscus often has its stereotyped ways of responding to almost any noxious stimuli; stomach cramps can result from stress, infection, and food poisoning alike. Moreover, the same general sort of pain, often described as a diffuse aching or burning, is shared in common by many different viscera.

Spatial Ambiguity

Interoception is reduced compared to surface perception not only in its qualitative range but in its spatial precision. Vision, audition, and touch allow me to locate stimuli to a fine degree. My fingers can tell apart pinpricks separated by only one to two millimeters. While other regions of the surface are less discriminating, I usually have little difficulty in locating cutaneous sensations. By way of contrast, visceral sensations are often vaguely situated with indistinct borders.[4] In my example, I experience midsection fullness and cramps, but there is no clear place where they begin or end, and no precise center.

Pain can suddenly localize when the sensitive membranes lining the visceral cavities become involved. But the inner organs themselves are in many instances simply incapable of registering localized events. Surgeons, for example, have found that they can cut the intestines in two without a conscious patient experiencing significant pain.[5] Like other viscera, the intestines primarily report generalized stimulations involving substantial portions of the organ.

The spatial ambiguity of the visceral depths is accentuated by the phenomenon of *referred pain*. A process taking place in one organ can experientially radiate to adjacent body areas or express itself in a distant location. Hence the pain of a heart attack may originate in the chest area but quickly spread down the left arm. This reflects embryological origins; sensation is referred to that level of the body the viscus occupied in the developing fetus before it descended, dragging nerves along, to its mature position. Thus, I may experience the pain where the organ used to be, not simply where it is now. An almost magical transfer of experience is effected along both spatial and temporal dimensions, weaving the inner body into an ambiguous space.[6]

Moreover, there are physical/phenomenal transfers between any vital organ and the body as a whole that further prohibit strict localization of visceral experience. Ricoeur refers to "this strange mixture of the local and the non-local" that is encountered in phenomena such as pain, hunger, thirst, and all vital needs.[7] As the example indicates, hunger is experienced not just in abdominal ache but as a heaviness in the limbs, a yearning in the mouth. The visceral organs sustain my body as a whole through processes of digestion, circulation, respiration, and excretion. Hence, when I manifest a visceral-based contentment or dysfunction, this is manifested everywhere and nowhere. A twinge in the finger is clearly located *there*. But hunger is a complex nexus of heaviness, exhaustion, conative urges, and discomforting sensations that, while gathering into nodes of crystallization, ambiguously inhabits the entirety of the corporeal field.

Spatiotemporal Discontinuity

The mysterious quality of our visceral space is based not only on such experiences but on all that is *not* experienced of our inner body. I have hitherto focused on what interoceptions we do have; they are marked by a limited qualitative range and a spatial ambiguity that together restrict our perceptual discriminations. Furthermore, as I will now address, there is a paucity of even such limited experiences.

Exteroception, at least during the waking state, manifests a certain spatiotemporal continuity. My eyes scan a visual world that is without sudden gaps or crevices. If I abandon one sense, perhaps closing my eyes, the other senses help to maintain the continuity of world. Similarly, proprioception traces out a completed sense of my surface body, allowing me to adjust every limb, every muscle, in appropriate motoric response to tasks. Though usually this sense is subliminal, I can close my eyes and proprioceptively hone in on the position, the level of tension or relaxation, in any region of the muscular body.

By way of contrast, the stream of interoceptive experience is marked by ineluctable discontinuities. In the above example, after eating the apple it largely disappeared from perception only to resurface in an experience of heartburn. This then faded away to silence, broken some time later by insistent cramps. This too passed. Finally, hours later I became aware of sensations from a new region signaling the need to defecate. But these are intermittent punctuations in a shroud of absence. Most of the intricate digestive process—its enzymatic secretions and peristaltic waves, its diffusions and active transports—proceeds without the possibility of conscious apprehension. This is equally true of circulation, respiration, thermal or fluid regulation. By far the greatest part of my vegetative processes lies submerged in impenetrable silence.

Causal relations are rendered uncertain by these spatiotemporal lacunae. I cannot be sure if my cramps are caused by an apple I previously ate, for this apple has, in the interim, disappeared from experience. Moments of discomfort are noted while the baseline of ordinary functioning is largely invisible. It is as if my eyes only reacted to flashes of blinding light, the rest of the time residing in darkness.

This darkness is never absolute. When I focus inward at even the quieter times I still find some vestigial sense of my midsection enveloped in a sort of sensory neutrality, neither full nor empty, pleasured nor in pain. And this vague aura is not devoid of meaning. It shows that any hunger or illness has subsided. The very absence of discomfort is tinged by a positivity.

Moreover, through a heightened focusing of attention, I can increase my awareness of visceral processes. Certain dim sensations that I had never noticed—the feeling of my pulsing blood, the depths of respiration, the subtler reactions of my stomach to different foods—can be brought into experience by conscious effort. As cultural variations show, a certain degree of visceral disappearance can be attributed to Western insensitivities and overcome by a systematic development of powers. The awareness of and control over the inner body exhibited by trained yogis has far surpassed what used to be thought possible in the West.

Yet even such achievements take place only within an overall context of experiential disappearance. The very need for highly specialized training is evidence of the perceptual reticence of our viscera as compared to the body surface. And just as it is possible to speak of nullpoints in relation to the surface body, the corporeal depths have their own phenomenological nullpoints. That is, there are visceral regions that are almost entirely insensitive. In focusing upon stomach and gut I have actually chosen two of the more loquacious organs. The kidney, gallbladder, bone marrow, spleen, yield far less interoceptively. The parenchyma of the liver, the alveolar tissue of the lung, are virtually without sensation.[8] Unlike the completed perception of the proprioceptive body, our inner body is marked by regional gaps, organs that although crucial for sustaining life, cannot be somesthetically perceived.[9]

We rarely thematize this sort of disappearance. Upon introspecting, I do not feel an emptiness in my body where my liver should be. This would make the absence into a presence-as-concealed hovering before my awareness. Rather, the absence of the liver parenchyma is so total that few would ever come to realize or remark upon it. Yet a medical mishap can suddenly awaken us to the significance of such bodily lacunae. The vast gaps in our inner perception may conceal potentially damaging processes until they are far advanced. For example, while I may feel pain once damage to the liver has progressed to the point of affecting its membranous capsule, the initial process can go unperceived. Similarly, hypertension is experientially hidden through much of its career.

As with my surface body, I can bring to bear upon these depth organs certain strategies of reflective observation. A blood sample can tell me a good deal about my liver function. Through a sphygmomanometer I can read off my blood pressure. I can look at an X ray of my lungs. I can even gaze through a colonoscope at the lumen and folds of my own colon. Such techniques enable me to gain knowledge concerning my viscera. Yet, as with my surface body, the absences that haunt my bodily depths are not effaced by these reflective maneuvers. Though I can visually observe my colon, its processes still elude experience from within. The magical power my body has to absorb water and electrolytes is not perceived as I gaze through the endoscope upon this furrowed, tubular space. The mystery of my body is only heightened by the very strangeness of the organ before me, its phenomenological noncoincidence with my body-as-lived.[10*]

Moreover, unlike the body surface, my inner organs tend to resist even these partial reflections. My viscera are ordinarily hidden away from the gaze by their location in the bodily depths. This aspect of withdrawal may seem contingent, resulting from a sheerly physical barrier rather than an existential principle. Yet this is to draw a false distinction; in the lived body, the physical and existential always intertwine.

The depth location of the viscera is no more contingent than the surface placement of the sensorimotor organs. Eye and hand could not perform their perceptual role unless they opened onto the external world. Thus, in order to perceive they must take their place among the perceptibles. They must be located at the body surface available to the gaze of myself and others. By way of contrast, my visceral organs, not constructed for ecstatic perception, disappear from the ranks of the perceived. I do not perceive *from* these organs; hence, they can hide beneath the body surface such that I do not perceive *to* them either. In fact, they require this seclusion just as the sensorimotor body requires exposure. My stomach, neither an organ of exteroception nor voluntary movement, could not screen the environment, secure appropriate foods, repel threats. It depends on a mediating surface, active and intelligent, to stand between it and the world, selecting what is needed for metabolic maintenance and protecting the viscus from hostile impacts. The hiddenness of vital organs, though frustrating at times of disease, is essential to healthy functioning.

Thus it is quite rare for the viscera to be exposed in life. This can happen, as in surgery, wartime injury, or violent accidents, yet these are pathological and dangerous occasions. Most commonly, the direct exposure of the inner organs implies or threatens the death of the person. Hence, as Foucault notes in *The Birth of the Clinic,* when nineteenth-century medicine made the direct perception of diseased organs an epistemological goal, the corpse, not the live patient, became the paradigmatic figure of truth. For the "anatomo-clinical" gaze, "that which hides and envelops, the curtain of night over truth, is, paradoxically, life; and death, on the contrary, opens up to the light of day the black coffer of the body."[11] While Foucault addresses this as a historical development, it manifests my phenomenological point; life itself is allied to a certain concealment, a withdrawal and protection of its vital center.

Visceral Motility

I have traced out a series of diverse ways in which the viscera disappear from awareness. My perception of the inner body is limited, ambiguous, and highly discontinuous. I will now turn to the topic of visceral motility where an equivalent principle can be seen at play.

In *The Primary World of Senses* Erwin Straus distinguishes between animal movement and that characteristic of inanimate things.[12] The latter yields to an analysis of mechanical forces. For example, we can understand the falling of a rock by referring to the sum total of the causal vectors acting upon it. Yet Straus attacks the physiological psychologists who would attempt to explain animal movement in the same way, treating locomotion as a summation of causal reflex arcs. He points out that it is first and foremost the entire animal that moves, not its motor units. And it moves because it is a being in relation to an experienced world, seeking desired goals, drawn to or repelled from a situation. I move my right arm to pick up an object of interest. The act must be understood in relation to its meaning, not as an amalgam of discrete muscle firings. This is as true of unplanned locomotion as it is of consciously chosen acts; unlike the falling rock, the dog who jumps away from an ongoing car still shows an existential grasp of the situation and an ability to respond to meanings.[13]

This distinction is crucial for opening up a genuinely phenomenological analysis of movement. Yet Straus, like most philosophers of embodiment, takes the activity of the surface motorium as paradigmatic for lived movement in general. I will turn attention instead to visceral motility. Such movement exhibits a structure of its own, sharing characteristics with and yet different from, both locomotion and inanimate movement. On the one hand, my vegetative processes are intertwined with my purposiveness, expressing moods and desires no less than does my surface body. If, for example, I am a chronically tense person, this may increase my stomach acid secretion. Yet, on the other hand, such a visceral function resists any attempt at direct command. My corporeal depths disappear not only from perception but relative to my structure of will and action.

The "It Can" and the "I Must"

To illustrate this point I will return to the phenomenological example given earlier. It began with a series of voluntary motor acts: walking in search of food, picking up and cutting an apple, taking a bite. All such movements arise out of the corporeal structure of the "I can" as described by Straus, Husserl, and Merleau-Ponty. I simply *can* walk, grasp, and bite, thereby bringing to fruition my gustatory project. This motor intentionality, as Merleau-Ponty points out, is prepersonal in an important sense. I have no explicit personal knowledge of how I physically perform such actions. Nor am I, for the most part, reflectively aware of my own "I-ness" while performing them. My attention is focused ecstatically on the perceptual scene or the desired object.

Yet, while prepersonal in such ways, the corporeal "I can" still speaks in the language of the first-person pronoun. There is no doubt that these are *my* actions. They relate to goals of personal significance, such as finding food to alleviate my hunger. I experience myself as personally responsible for such acts. When my desires change or someone requests it, I can alter or terminate the activity at will.

However, once the bolus of food is swallowed it enters a very different volitional space. Scientific investigations have shown that an intricate series of movements ensue. The epiglottis folds over, the esophagus shudders with a peristaltic wave, and the gastroesophageal sphincter loosens its grip. Then stomach and gut take over with their intricate rhythms of churning, secreting, contracting, each to their own measured and idiosyncratic pace. Yet such movements are not experienced as within the "I can" of personal mastery. I do not feel a sense of guiding or controlling these processes. Once initiated by my act of eating, the rest proceeds *automatically;* etymologically the word *automatic* means "self-moving."[14]

We might then say that this level of the body exhibits an "it can" more that an "I can." It (be it heart, kidney, or lung) can accomplish its vital tasks without my awareness or volition. As Ricoeur writes:

> In effect, it is extraordinary that life functions in me without me, that the multiple hormone balances which science reveals constantly reestablish themselves within me without my help. This is extraordinary because at a certain level of my existence I no longer appear to myself as a *task,* as a project. I am a *problem resolved* as though by a greater wisdom than myself. This wisdom is a nourishing one: when I have eaten, it is not up to me to make the food into myself and grow on it. It is a wisdom of movement: the circulation of my blood and the beating of my heart do not depend upon me.[15]

For Descartes this strange power is explained via reference to the ontological duality of the self. Whereas desired actions are brought about directly by the soul, movements such as eating and breathing, "which we make without our will contributing thereto,"[16] proceed purely from the mechanical body. While pointing up the phenomenological shift between the "I can" and the "it can," this dualism fails to account for intermediate levels of volition and the profound interconnection of the sensorimotor and the visceral.

Aristotle, alternatively, has recourse to the notion of a multiplicity of souls or powers of soul. We share with other animals appetitive, sensory, and locomotive powers, and we are set apart by the thinking part of the soul. Yet we have as well a nutritive or reproductive soul that we hold in common with all living things, plants included. While ultimately incapable of separate existence in man, the nutritive soul thus has a quasi independence, proceeding without the direct use of appetitive or rational powers.

Soul in Aristotle's terminology is not the immaterial substance to which Descartes refers. Rather, it is the very actuality, end, and essence of a body possessed potentially of life.[17] The "ensouled" body is precisely the body as living and lived. In referring to the multiple powers of the soul, Aristotle thus recognizes what would here be termed the multileveled nature of the lived body. This body includes not only ecstatic functions but visceral or "nutritive" powers that unfold in an autonomous fashion.

Compared to the ecstatic level, the range of visceral motility, like that of interoception, is limited in several ways. Organs of the surface are constructed to engage in a wide variety of actions; the mouth, for example, not only eats but breathes, talks, sings, whistles, lubricates, cries out, spits. By contrast the motor possibilities of the viscera are restricted and preordained. Each organ plays its determined role, the lung in respiration, the stomach in food storage and breakdown, etc.[18] Yet what the "it can" can do is clearly sufficient. The surface body, turned outward to the world, must have a motoric plasticity, an ability to respond to various and unpredictable challenges. But the objects with which the viscera must cope have already been preselected, filtered, and channeled by the surface. Barring mishap, what reaches the lung will be air, the stomach, food or drink. Their fixed motile patterns will thus be adequate. The preordained style of visceral activity depends upon the plasticity of the surface.

The converse is true as well. Because I can trust my vegetative body to manage the repetitive assimilations and excretions, I am freed up to focus upon novel tasks. If I had to remember to breathe or had to stage-manage each phase of my digestion, there would be little time left for other activities. The surface body is liberated by such automaticities.

Yet this automatic level also places calls upon me, guiding and limiting my choices. I must tailor my actions to visceral rhythms. Buytendijk addresses this with the example of hunger:

> As with all vital modes of being . . . hunger arises from our bodily subjectivity as a power which rules us personally, locks us in and at whose mercy we are, as long as it lasts.[19]

Thus, the visceral body gives rise not only to an "it can" but to an "I must." I must eat, breathe, excrete, drink, sleep, at certain times and in certain ways to mollify inner demands.[20] My personal subjectivity can choose how to fulfill such biological needs, eating one food rather than another. But it does not assert a final autonomy. I may temporarily postpone a meal, but if I engage in prolonged self-starvation, this will eventually threaten my life. When the personal subject seeks to overcome the vegetative "I must," it is the subject who is ultimately overcome. For these vegetative processes exhibit a "foreign-mineness";[21] while seemingly Other to the self, they are nonetheless integral to the self's existence.

The "I Cannot"

The foreignness of this inner body—the automaticity of the "it can," the demanding character of the "I must"—ultimately refers back to a structure of personal inability. I will term this the "I cannot." I cannot act from my inner organs in the way I do from my surface musculature. Though I can lift my arm without any problem, I cannot in the same way choose to secrete a little more bile or accelerate my digestion. The "magical" sway I have over my own body that Merleau-Ponty describes[22] thus refers primarily to the body surface. The depths involve an even deeper sorcery extending beyond my domain. As Lewis Thomas observes:

> If I were informed tomorrow that I was in direct communication with my liver, and could now take over, I would become deeply depressed. I'd sooner be told, forty thousand feet over Denver, that the 747 jet in which I had a coach seat was now mine to operate as I pleased; at least I would have the hope of bailing out, if I could find a parachute and discover quickly how to open a door. Nothing would save me and my liver, if I were in charge. For I am, to face the facts squarely, considerably less intelligent than my liver. I am, moreover, constitutionally unable to make hepatic decisions, and I prefer not be obliged to, ever. I would not be able to think of the first thing to do.[23]

The curious nature of this "I cannot" can be correlated with the data of physiology. The surface body is covered with striated or voluntary muscle, connected by motor neurons directly to the central nervous system. This is not the case with the smooth muscle (and cardiac muscle) of the viscera. The contractile level of such muscle is modulated by the endocrine organs and the autonomic nervous system. The digestive tract, for example, while utilizing striated muscle at its extremes, is surrounded by smooth muscle from two-thirds of the way down the esophagus until the anorectal juncture. Such transitions, visible to the scientist from without, correspond roughly to transitions in experience from within. Once the apple is swallowed it passes out of my domain of action, its intricate passage and absorption governed by the "it can." Only when the stage of defecation is reached, do we reclaim a measure of personal command. We have resurfaced to the level of the "I can."

Thus, the inner body manifests a motoric withdrawal similar to that vis-à-vis perception. Just as the viscera retreat from conscious experience, so they recede from volitional control. Moreover, these two forms of reticence are biologically/existentially intertwined. My ability to make exteroceptive discriminations is significant only because I can act discriminatingly; once having perceived the difference between things, I can choose to eat this rather than that, to pursue one object and flee another.[24] This choice is no longer available once objects have been internalized. Since my range of purposeful action has then effectively ended, a detailed experience of the visceral space would be useless. In the words of the neurophysiologist Sherrington:

> Once through the maw, the morsel is, we know by introspection, under normal circumstances lost for consciousness. . . . The significant point is that the object has passed into such a relation with the surface of the organism that 'conation' is no longer of advantage. The naive notion that when we have eaten and drunk we have *fed* is justified *practically*. No *effort* can help us to incorporate the food further. . . . It is significant that all direct psychical accompaniment of the reaction ceases abruptly at this very point.[25]

The "I cannot" of visceral action and perception are mutually correlative and form a unified system.

Indirection and the Medical Field

The previous discussion has revolved around a central point; one's inner body withdraws from direct perception and control. However, I have yet to address certain *indirect* modes of self-apprehension. I can indirectly perceive and modify my own vegetative functions through the intermediary of the surface body. Insofar as this is a primary mode of relating to the inner body, it merits a separate, if brief, discussion. In so doing, I will focus upon medical examples to suggest the import of visceral disappearance relative to this field.

As noted earlier, all self-perception involves a divergence between observer and observed. The eye from which I see never quite coincides with its mirror image. This surface self-perception might be termed *direct but noncoincident.* While the eye is directly visible to itself in the mirror, there is a noncoincidence between the "from" and the "to" perspective.

In terming much of visceral apprehension *indirect,* I refer to the advent of another, surplus form of mediation. This occurs when directly-given perceptions are interpreted as disclosing processes themselves unperceived. In this case, visceral functions unavailable to interoception are indirectly inferred from surface states. Similarly, I can exert control by indirection. In situations where I have no direct command over visceral processes, I can indirectly influence them through my purposive acts.

All vegetative processes depend to some degree upon exchanges with the environment. They then must surface, and at such points of initiation and termination become available to the surface "I can." While I cannot perceive most of the digestive process itself, I can see what I eat and later excrete. From this I can indirectly infer a great deal concerning my digestion; I know what is being digested, and when, and how successfully. I can as well manifest control at such points, choosing what to eat or when to defecate. I cannot simply will my stomach and gut to better perform. But I can indirectly assist these organs by avoiding certain foods or, in the case of illness, swallowing the proper medications.

Thus, reversing the usual phenomenal field, vegetative processes involve a central disappearance surrounded by clear and distinct horizons. They surface primarily at their periphery to sensorimotor command. Different functions are characterized by differing ratios of surface to depth. For example, digestion, as a lengthy spatiotemporal circuit, is buried for long stretches from the sensorimotor self. Respiration, involving surface exchanges renewed several times a minute, is far more accessible. I can feel the air entering my nostrils. I proprioceptively sense my chest and abdomen expanding and can utilize appropriate muscles to change the rate or quality of breath.[26] Nevertheless, in any visceral process there remains a central absence that can only be indirectly known. The actual air exchange in the lung's alveolar tissue is unavailable to direct awareness and control.

Visceral functions surface not just at orifices of initiation and termination but at multiple points along the way. My arteries approach close enough to the skin in several places for my pulse to be externally palpable. I thus gain an indirect reading of my heart function. Then too, a circulatory failure may surface as a bluish tinge or a "clubbing" at the fingernails or as palpable edema in the legs.

Such signs are often utilized in medical diagnosis. The physician is a hermeneut, reading the text of the surface body for what it has to say about corporeal depths.[27] The ambiguities of this tale, the inferential and uncertain nature of diagnosis, can never be fully effaced. This is an offshoot, to a degree, of visceral disappearance. The same can be said of the limitations and difficulties attending medical therapeutics. Any attempt at conscious, rational control over the viscera must seek to overcome their natural autonomy. The doctor thus labors to see what cannot be seen, to command what is ordinarily beyond command.

The doctor is aided in this attempt by technological incorporations. Via endoscopes, stethoscopes, X rays, needles, the patient's bodily depths are made available to the doctor's sensorimotor province. The doctor has artificially supplemented his or her embodiment, enabling a "gaze" that heretofore was impossible. In addition to transforming the physician's embodiment, the patient's own body may be altered. A surgical exposure, for example, brings the patient's depths temporarily up to the surface (or permanently, as in the case of some colostomies). The viscera are thus rendered visible and susceptible to manipulation. Such direct interventions are still "indirect" in a phenomenological sense. The patient is utilizing the body of another as an indirect conduit of perception and control.

Up until now the surfacing of visceral circuitry through defined points or methods has been emphasized: orifices, pulses, surgeries, and the like. Yet this intertwining of surface and depth characterizes the entire body to a degree. My sensorimotor functions are highly dependent upon my visceral processes. As discussed, hunger is not just in my stomach but pervades my mouth, my muscles, my mood. It is everywhere, manifesting as exhaustion and craving, irritability and impatience. I can thus indirectly experience the visceral through its effects on the entire corporeal field. And since my corporeal field is always in relation to a world, the visceral saturates my environment as well. Carolina Maria de Jesus provides an example of this as she describes the resolution of a prolonged hunger:

> What a surprising effect food has on our organisms. Before I ate, I saw the sky, the trees, and the birds all yellow, but after I ate, everything was normal to my eyes. . . . I was able to work better. My body stopped

weighing me down. . . . I started to smile as if I was witnessing a beautiful play.[28]

The world itself shifts with a shift in the visceral.

Correlatively, a change in the world or my relation to it can swiftly
change my visceral state. If I encounter or even think about a distressing
scene, my heart beats faster and certain blood vessels constrict. If I start
running in place another set of cardiovascular changes ensue. I can thus
indirectly manage the visceral through controlling my conscious acts or
environment. This principle is highly significant in the treatment and
prevention of disease. We can alter our visceral functioning and thus
our health history by reducing environmental stress, ridding our air
and water of pollutants, choosing to exercise and eat properly, avoiding
noxious substances such as nicotine, and even through embracing positive emotions and thoughts.[29] Increasingly recognized within orthodox
medicine, such interventions have long been at the core of "holistic" and
"behavioral" approaches. Such treatments, no less than the conventional
use of pills or surgery, are still indirect in my technical sense. If I give up
cigarettes and take up jogging in order to avoid a heart attack, I am
employing my surface body to indirectly transform the visceral.

This is not to say that all visceral control must be mediated and indirect. While it was once assumed that autonomic functions were necessarily involuntary, biomedical research over the last twenty-five years
has challenged that presumption. It was found that visceral processes,
not merely those of the skeletal muscles, could be controlled through
operant conditioning. Animals and humans exhibited the ability to alter functions such as heart rate and rhythm, blood pressure, vasomotor
responses, and salivation.[30] Experiments further suggested that these
visceral changes need not be mediated through the surface motorium
but may be elicited independently or as part of a general skeletal-vis-
ceral pattern.[31] On the clinical front, such research has given rise to
biofeedback techniques whereby individuals are taught to lower their
blood pressure, control cardiac arrythmias, avoid migraine headaches,
etc.[32] These developments have also increased scientific interest in and
research on modes of visceral control exercised in other cultures. Most
famously, trained yogis have shown the ability to markedly slow heart
rate and metabolic function or perform highly specific alterations, such
as lowering the temperature of one hand while raising it in the other.[33]

However, even in such cases, the principle of indirection plays a part.
To perform such feats, the yogi must undergo extensive training and
often makes use of "surface" functions, such as mantras, visual images,
and breath control. This indirection is clearly present in the case of biofeedback training for visceral processes. An internal function, such as

blood pressure, is monitored electronically and "fed back" to the subject in the form of exteroceptive stimuli, often light or sound. Once made available in this form, the subject can learn to control what before was involuntary. Self-knowledge and self-command are thus achieved through technological mediation; what was depth is artificially made to surface.

Depth Disappearance

My analysis of the inner body has been diverse and detailed. Yet there is a common principle unifying the various discussions. A mode of disappearance is at work. A large segment of my visceral processes simply do not appear to conscious perception. My apprehension is mainly indirect or involving limited, ambiguous interoceptions. Moreover, visceral processes disappear from my field of action. I do not for the most part command my own vital functions but rely upon their automaticities. What influence I exert is largely through indirect pathways.

I will term this visceral withdrawal a *depth disappearance* to distinguish it from the sorts of disappearance characteristic of the surface body. For, as I will suggest, the operative principle is not merely an extension of that involved in focal and background disappearance. Depth disappearance operates in other ways. The notion of depth indicates not only a physical site but a genuinely distinct phenomenological dimension.

As previously discussed, the surface body tends to disappear from thematic awareness precisely because it is that *from* which I exist in the world. Directed ecstatically outward, my organs of perception and motility are themselves transparent at the moment of use. This is the principle of focal disappearance. The intentional arc has a telos that carries attention outward, away from its bodily points of origin.

Conversely, the viscera disappear precisely because they are displaced from this arc. They are that part of the body which we do *not* use to perceive or act upon the world in a direct sense. For example, my liver is not the point of origin of a projective sensory field. It is ordinarily devoid of sensation. Its disappearance is thus not a function of ecstasis. Rather, my liver recedes beneath the reach of my personal awareness and control. In contrast to the ecstatic body, which "stands out," I will term this the body *recessive;* etymologically, to re-cede means to "go or fall back." The body not only projects outward in experience but falls back into unexperienceable depths.

Because ecstatic organs remain part of the experiential arc, though usually marginal to consciousness, they can be thematized in a variety of ways. If my hand reaches out to touch an object, I can, via an attentional shift, experience the stream of sensations as within my hand. Moreover, I can touch one hand with another.

As we have seen, the recessive body is more difficult to thematize. Just as I cannot perceive or act from the viscera, neither can I, for the most part, perceive or act to them. Buried within the bodily depths, my viscera resist my reflective gaze and physical manipulation. To be in depth disappearance is ordinarily to recede from the arc of personal involvement as a whole, neither subject nor object of direct engagement. This is true as well of objects incorporated into depth disappearance. The apple, once swallowed, largely vanishes from my conscious perception and control.

This is not to imply that depth disappearance is absolute. All forms of corporeal absence are intertwined with modes of presence. As discussed, there is some perception of the viscera, albeit reduced, and several modes of indirect awareness and command. Nevertheless, there is a foreignness to the inner body that in many ways surpasses that of the surface. I would not even recognize my own viscera if they were somehow presented to my gaze. I would stand in the presence of something uncanny and alien—could such organs really be inside of me? The repulsion we may feel in the face of our own feces or vomitus is an expression of this alienness-from-within.

In describing a region of the body that disappears not via its participation in but its withdrawal from the ecstatic sensorimotor arc, I may seem to be recapitulating the structure of background disappearance. As discussed, this term refers to the experiential absence of parts of the body functionally put out of play or used in a manner irrelevant or merely supportive to the main focus of activity. If, for example, I am fully engaged in listening to a concert, my closed eyes, my stilled legs, are enfolded in a background disappearance. No longer perceiving or acting from such organs, they temporarily withdraw from awareness.

Yet, these surface organs at the next moment may be employed in a focal manner. I can always get up and open my eyes. The functioning of legs and eyes remains within the province of the "I can"; it is my projects that have put them out of play and can summon them back to life. While currently reticent, such organs are still part of the corporeal field of possibilities through which I encounter the world. Background and focal disappearance thus stand in a relation of potential reversibility similar to the background and focus of a perceptual field.

Depth disappearance opens up a third dimension. Unlike the surface organ in background disappearance, a viscus is largely irreversible with corporeal foci. It cannot be summoned up for personal use, turned ec-statically upon the world. Its recessiveness is not simply the function of a current gestalt but of an innate resistance.

In understanding the relation of the three forms of disappearance it is useful to reintroduce the concept of the complemental series. I have defined a complemental series as the emergence of a phenomenon from the balanced operation of two etiological factors, where the rising of one is necessarily linked to the other's decline. I have discussed how the ab-sence of the surface body can be accounted for via the complemental series constituted by focal and background disappearance.

Now a second complemental series operative in the distinction be-tween body surface and depth can be recognized. Experience attests to a certain forgetting of the body in general. Yet the causative factors at play differ at different physical/phenomenal levels. If we were to imagine ourselves descending through corporeal layers, we would see a gradual shift from those modes of disappearance characteristic of the sen-sorimotor "I" to that form which typifies the anonymous depths. Sur-face organs are forgotten via their structural role, focal or background, in the ecstatic arc, while the viscera recede beneath the reach of this arc. The body disappears both as a seat of consciousness and as the site of an unconscious vitality.

Our lack of conscious awareness and control vis-à-vis aspects of the self has formed a recurrent theme of postrationalist thought. The self, it is realized, is in many ways foreign to itself, leading to the postulation of an "unconscious." Yet paradoxes arise when this notion is reified and mentalized, as if it were a second consciousness hidden from the first. Merleau-Ponty refers us back to a bodily unconscious, rooted in our sen-sorimotor response to the world.[34] Prior to explicit acts of positing, our body grasps multiple, ambiguous meanings that elude articulation and conceptual grasp. There is thus an indeterminacy, a horizonality, an un-consciousness, adhering to the sensorimotor self. My analysis does not dispute but supplements the Merleau-Pontian reading. For I have point-ed toward a further visceral dimension to the body unconscious.[35*] Sexuality lies rooted in a deep reproductive circuitry with its own cycles and automaticities. Emotions are mediated by the autonomic nervous system and internal hormonal shifts. Belonging at least partially to the visceral, these functions partake in its depth disappearance. We do not fully know from whence our desires and moods arise. Moreover, as most of us are painfully aware, they often resist the commands of the egoic self.

While a complemental series is articulated via its two poles, it gives rise to an entire range of intermediate phenomena. This is true of the series constituted by body surface and depth.[36] Desire may be stimulated by a hormonal buildup or by a lover's seductive glance. As I will address in chapter 5, desires and emotions involve an intertwining of visceral and ecstatic features. There are, as well, anatomical structures that particularly exhibit the intermediate mode. For example, the parietal membranes that line the visceral cavities can be the source of sharply localized sensations. Though buried in the bodily depths, these structures are innervated by spinal nerve fibers that penetrate inward from the body surface. Then too, there is the brain. Encased within the skull, its neurons are yet derived from embryological surface tissue. Moreover, the brain is the functional regulator both of vegetative states and conscious volitional processes. As I will discuss in chapter 4, this organ is the very paradigm of surface-depth intertwining.

Ultimately this relationship of exchange and intertwining characterizes all parts of the body, though one or another mode of function may predominate. The visceral depths always participate in ecstasis. As was shown, a hunger or hormonal mood colors the entire world. Vegetative needs motivate our projects and selectively channel our attention. Thus, in the broadest sense we act and experience from the visceral no less than from the sensorimotor body. Conversely, the surface body participates in depth disappearance. Even the most "transparent" sense organ has tissue layers and physiological functions that lie beneath the reach of one's own experience. Moreover, the surface body has aspects that resist personal control. I do not heal my scars, build my eyes, supervise the growth or loss of my hair. While it is within my province to move my hand, it was not I that first posited fingers, nor can I prevent their arthritic aging. Even my own hand movements elude control when motor reflexes come into play. Just as the visceral can surface to volition, as through biofeedback or yogic techniques, so surface motility can sink into the realm of the automatic.[37]

Hence, I inhabit one body, ecstatic-recessive in its entirety. Each organ both projects outward and recedes inward, eluding the self bidirectionally. I have heretofore emphasized the contrast between different regions in order to clarify distinct modes of body absence and show how their varying dominance serves to define a phenomenological anatomy. In everyday experience the inner body is characterized primarily by its recession from awareness and control. The body surface, conversely, is lived out primarily through ecstasis. Yet this contrast does not constitute a new dualism. It only serves to highlight the limit points of a complemental series that embraces interfusion, exchanges, and intermediate modes.

Temporal Depths

I have arrived at the structure of depth disappearance through a spatio-functional analysis of the body. That is, I have examined regions of the body distinguished by their locale, functional properties, and associated experiential modes. Yet, as previously discussed, a phenomenological anatomy cannot remain static in form. The body is not a grouping of fixed features but a being in process undergoing historical development and cyclic transformations. My spatialized analysis must again be supplemented by adequate recognition of the temporal. *Depth* can then be understood not simply in terms of the inner organs but as referring to temporal phases of embodiment. To clarify this point I will briefly examine the cyclic phenomenon of sleep, as well as the historical birth process from which each one of us emerged.

Sleep

Erwin Straus writes:

> Awakeness is a primitive fact. It is the foundation upon which is erected the human world, in the praxis of life as in theoretical insight, in its interhuman intercourse as in its individual and common history.[38]

I can write this work and you can read it only because we share a waking commitment to the world. Being awake is the precondition for outer-directed perception, motility, and social engagement. In examining the ways in which we disregard our bodies, I have thus hitherto assumed the waking subject.

But my own body also disappears when I am asleep in a way more thorough than any yet encountered. Sleep is precisely a form of withdrawal from experience. When attending to the phenomenon of sleep, philosophers and psychologists have often focused on the dreaming state, for this is the portion of sleep that most restores an experiential process. However, a dream is only made possible by a preliminary severance from waking involvements. It is this severance, this loss of consciousness to the world, that is shared to some degree by all phases of sleep.

A phenomenology of falling asleep provides a clue to the mode of disappearance involved. Just as I cannot will my visceral processes, I cannot directly will my sleep. My limbs grow heavy, eyes flutter shut, perceptual and intellectual alertness slip away. While I can intervene, shaking myself awake, I cannot force sleep upon myself. It involves a "letting happen," a giving up of resistance to a call placed upon me. It is when I decide to fall asleep and set about this with a vengeance that insomnia strikes.

As with visceral processes, what I do not directly control I can indirectly influence. I close the door, dim the lights, quiet my sensorimotor body, one by one loosening the ties that bind me to the world. Merleau-Ponty writes:

> As the faithful, in the Dionysian mysteries, invoke the god by miming scenes from his life, I call up the visitation of sleep by imitating the breathing and posture of the sleeper.[39]

But this state is only an imitation, not an actualization of sleep. As I lie awake my ears still hear stray noises. My limbs, while quieted, remain within my motor control. My body is in background disappearance, put out of active play, but still available to will and world.

When sleep overcomes me I enter something deeper. My ears become all but deaf to the sounds around me, my eyes not merely shut but vacated. My limbs lie beyond the range of my volition. This then is a mode of depth disappearance now enfolding the body in its entirety. The body is no longer ecstatic, that from which I perceive and act, but a being recessed from my command and awareness. As I no longer perceive from this body, neither can I perceive to it. This is even more true than in the case of my internal organs, for those remained accessible through a limited interoception. In deep sleep, interoception, proprioception, exteroception—all recede. My own sleeping body is one thing I will never directly see. Where "it" is, "I," as conscious, perceiving subject, necessarily am not.

As with the visceral organs, modes of indirect perception remain. Upon awakening in the morning I can infer from the light outside, the shape of my bedclothes, and my current bodily feelings something about the length and quality of my sleep. Or I can learn of it indirectly through another. I am the one person who will never be able to hear myself snore, but my wife will describe it in no uncertain terms.

Indeed, while I cannot perceive my sleeping body, another can, more easily than they could my internal organs. Yet as in that case, the withdrawal of a body region from ecstatic engagement involves a certain absence from others as well as from oneself. In order to fall asleep I sever my social and perceptual involvements, generally retreating to a dark and quiet space. As a result, most of the world has only seen my body-when-awake.

The sleeping body thus partakes of all aspects of depth disappearance. It disappears from perception and command, from self and Other, as a result of its withdrawal from the sensorimotor circuit. The complemental series constituted by body surface and depth here exhibits a temporal dimension. I oscillate between the depth disappearance of sleep and the mixed modes characteristic of the waking self.[40]

A complemental series, by definition, embraces a range of intermediate phenomena. Between deep sleep and alert wakefulness lie a variety of transitional states through which I cyclically move. The dream state is a good example; there is a vivid flow of perceptual experience, yet coupled with a recessed embodiment.[41] Then too, there is the twilight state where one is "half-asleep," suspended between ecstasis and recession, the "I can" and the "I cannot." Movements are laborious, sounds heard dimly as if from far away. In light sleep, recessiveness has clearly gained the upper hand, but there remains a sensitivity to outer stimuli. Even in moderately deep sleep, people respond with EEG bursts when a meaningful sound, such as their name, is whispered. One's intentional threads to the world are never fully severed, not even in the deepest sleep, for a strong enough stimuli will always seize one back.

Yet, in deep sleep, we discover the radical anonymity of natural existence. Nightly, I give my life over to those vegetative processes that form but a circumscribed region of my day-body. Surface functions all but abandoned, I become a creature of depth, lost in respiration, digestion, and circulation. My experiential world rests upon the restorative powers of this unconscious being. I can surface for only a limited time before requiring resubmergence in the impersonal.

Birth

Each waking day is double-horizoned by sleep. Yet there is an even more global horizon to sleeping and waking alike, to all ecstatic and recessive phenomena: life itself. The precondition of all my experience is that I have come into life and hence have undergone a gestation and birth. Yet this point of origination is marked by ineradicable absence. Ricoeur writes:

> My birth is the beginning of my life: in it I was placed, once and for all, into the world, and posed in being before I was able to posit any act voluntarily. Yet this central event to which I refer in dating all the events of my life leaves no memory. I am always *after* my birth—in a sense analogous to that of being always *before* my death. I find myself alive—I am already born. Furthermore, nothing shows me that there had been a beginning of myself: my birth is precisely what remains hidden from my consciousness.[42]

Birth thus constitutes a temporal nullpoint. The central event from which all my experience radiates is itself hidden from direct awareness.

As with the other nullpoints discussed, this absence is not merely a de facto occurrence but essential to the structure of the lived body. In the words of Merleau-Ponty:

> The fact that my earliest years lie behind me like an unknown land is not attributable to any chance lapse in memory, or any failure to think back adequately: there is nothing to be known in these unexplored lands. For example, in pre-natal existence, nothing was perceived, and therefore there is nothing to recall. There was nothing but the raw material and adumbration of a natural self and a natural time.[43]

While Merleau-Ponty exaggerates in saying the fetus perceives nothing, it does belong primarily to the natural and not the personal sphere. Like the body asleep, the fetus is a recessive being, dwelling largely in metabolic anonymity.

This, then, is another form of depth disappearance. I do not perceive or act from my embryonic body. In the earliest stages of gestation, my surface sensorimotor functions are still undeveloped. As I do not perceive from this body, neither could I perceive to it, leaving a nullpoint in experience and memory.

As with other forms of depth disappearance, this recessive body is mainly available through indirection. My very being alive refers me back to a necessary, though elusive, point of origin. Its traces are imprinted upon my body in the form of a navel. I can see photographs of my infancy, extending my current vision through incorporated technologies. Others can inform me whether I was a cute or ugly baby and tell me the circumstances of my birth. Indeed, most of my knowledge of my gestation and early life comes through the mediation of others.

Yet, as we have seen, depth disappearance also fosters an intersubjective withdrawal. Just as the vital organs must recede from the world, and the sleeper from social and perceptual engagements, so the fetus must be enfolded away. Prior to the maturation of sensorimotor powers one is dependent upon the protection and nutrition provided by another's body. Hidden within a womb, one is largely invisible to the gaze of others, even that of one's own mother.

For gestation involves her body as well in a depth disappearance. The mysterious process of conception and implantation takes place out of the range of her apprehension and will. One's parents indirectly initiated the process via the conjugation of surface bodies. But once initiated, an impersonal viscerality takes over, guiding life through its intricate development. The early stages are largely imperceptible—hence the frequent question, "Am I pregnant or not?" The mother experiences early gestational processes indirectly through its global effects on her body: nausea, food cravings, and the like. Later there is an interoceptive experience of the fetus's movements. One can even feel with one's hands its head pressing against the abdominal wall. Yet, as with all visceral processes, such perceptions are highly limited, traces of a vast invisible realm.

When the baby is born there is a sudden *excorporation* from depth disappearance. The movement of incorporation, as with skills or tools or the ingestion of food, is here reversed. What was part of the body is now made extrinsic. Yet while birth terminates depth disappearance in relation to the maternal body, it does not fully do so in relation to the child's. For the first time the infant body gains a full surface, interfacing directly with the world rather than through the mother's mediating flesh. Sensorimotor threads must now be woven to replace the umbilical threads that hitherto sustained life. But this development of an ecstatic body, begun in fetal life, is as yet incomplete. It will come to fruition only through a series of environmental challenges and the gradual mye-linization of nerves. The human infant is born several months premat-ure compared to other mammals; its oversized head would be unable later to traverse the birth canal. For months after birth we thus remain largely visceral in character, devoted to eating, excretion, and sleep.

Hence, this body is still dominated by depth disappearance. The newborn does not for the most part act from the "I can" toward desired goals. Command over bodily functions takes time to develop. Nor can she or he be said to have mastered perceptual ecstasis. Psychological theorists, such as Mahler[44] and Winnicott,[45] agree that the newborn in-fant does not yet distinguish between its body and that of the mother, between sensations of internal and external origin. There is, in Mahler's terms, a "symbiotic" phase that precedes the differentiation of self and Other. The projective structure of perception, whereby I experience bodily sensations as disclosing an outer and separate world, is not estab-lished until some months after birth. Only then can the infant begin to perceive to its body as a defined entity. Through the "mirror stage"[46] and other such perceptual reflections, a body-image gradually coalesces. The shift from a visceral to a sensorimotor and self-conscious body is an ongoing task for the first few years of life.

Hence birth itself is but an intermediate phenomenon in yet another form of the complemental series. I historically progress from the pure depth disappearance that characterizes embryonic life to the various forms of disappearance in the body matured. In the depths of my past I encounter that same viscerality that resides in the depths of my inner body and the depths of sleep. The conscious, active "I" is in every direc-tion outrun.

The Flesh and Blood

In closing my discussion of depth, I will situate this concept in relation to the work of Merleau-Ponty. This brief excursus will serve two functions. First, the rich web of concepts and terms supplied by Merleau-Ponty will prove useful for summarizing my own findings. Indeed, his work on embodiment has formed the inspiration and source of many of the ideas found here. However, there is a second reason for turning explicitly to Merleau-Ponty; I will suggest that a recognition of depth points out an incompletion in his project. His valorization of the lived body goes hand in hand with his thesis of the "primacy of perception."[47] Yet the former notion is not coextensive with the latter. The lived body, as we have seen, is far more than a perceiver/perceived. Beneath the sensorimotor surface lies the anonymous strata of the visceral, a prenatal history, the body asleep. Within the *Phenomenology of Perception,* Merleau-Ponty makes passing reference to such dimensions of embodiment but never allows their full significance to emerge.

In the working notes collected in *The Visible and the Invisible* he criticizes his earlier work "due to the fact that in part I retained the philosophy of 'consciousness.' "[48] He now seeks to escape the limits of an analysis based on intentionality and subjective awareness. Commentators such as Gary Madison[49] have emphasized the crucial shift this effects in his project, the divergence between the early and later Merleau-Ponty. If space is to be made for the unconscious depths, we might then search for it in *The Visible and the Invisible,* his culminating, though unfinished work. It is to this volume that I now turn my attention.

Flesh: The Chiasmatic Structure

In *The Visible and the Invisible,* Merleau-Ponty seeks to bring to "ontological explicitation" (*VI,* 183) his previous phenomenological studies. He thus supplants his terminology of the lived body with the ontological notion of "flesh" (*la chair*). Flesh belongs neither to the subject nor world exclusively. It is a primal "element" (*VI,* 139) out of which both are born in mutual relation. It cannot then be conceived of as mind or as material substance. Rather, the "flesh" is a kind of circuit, a "coiling over of the visible upon the visible" (*VI,* 140), which traverses me but of which I am not the origin.

Merleau-Ponty gives specificity to this notion by articulating a series of "chiasmatic" relations, "intertwinings" (*entrelacs*) that characterize the flesh. Just as the three-dimensionality of visual space depends upon the optic chiasm blending fibers from both eyes, so the world leaps out of a "chiasm" between subject and object, my vision and that of others, perception and language. I will briefly explore these chiasmatic links, arguing that they are insufficient to do full justice to the visceral.

Because the human body is an *"exemplar sensible"* (*VI*, 135)—a structure in which is captured and exhibited the general structure of the world—Merleau-Ponty begins his analysis of flesh by examining the lived body. Utilizing the example of one hand touching another, he shows that the body can play the role both of perceiver and perceived, subject and object. It is as if the body had "two outlines," "two sides," "two leaves" (*VI*, 136–37). As discussed in my chapter 1, these never quite coincide. Insofar as I touch my right hand, I capture it as material object but no longer experience from it as the toucher. There is according to Merleau-Ponty, a "divergence" (*écart*), a "fission" that stops the body as subject and object from quite merging. Yet this is an identity-in-difference.[50] The two sides of the body are not ontologically separate categories as Sartre might have it, the subject's absolute nothingness, the object's plenitude of being. My hand could not touch unless it itself were tangible, installed in the same world as its objects. The lived body is necessarily chiasmatic, a perceiver/perceived.

This intertwining thus characterizes the body's relationship to its world. As perceiver I am necessarily made of the same flesh as the things I confront. I could not experience a world whose essential properties were radically discontinuous from mine. Correlatively, for Merleau-Ponty, the world is always a world-as-perceived (*VI*, 131), not a scientific object or a thing-in-itself. "The flesh of the world is of the Being-seen, i.e. is a Being that is *eminently percipi*" (*VI*, 250).

The full reality of this sensible world arises not simply from the power of sight, or any single such mode, but from the mutual reference and intertwining of all forms of perception. "There is double and crossed situating of the visible in the tangible and of the tangible in the visible; the two maps are complete, and yet they do not merge into one" (*VI*, 134). This book as you experience it is a chiasmatic product of both vision and touch. Such an intertwining of sensory worlds can occur only because my body is an intertwining, not just of perceiver and perceived but of different *ways* of perceiving. "My synergic body . . . assembles into a cluster the 'consciousnesses' adherent to its hands, to its eyes, by an operation that is in relation to them lateral, transversal" (*VI*, 141).

If my own body is already a prereflective synergy of different consciousnesses, it is not hard for me to understand the arising of consciousness in another's body. Here the flesh articulates into another chiasmatic relation: that which links me to other perceivers. Our perspectives on the world, though never quite coinciding, intertwine in mutual validation. The reality of the world is secured via its presence to other perspectives than my own. Even my own body is brought to full fruition only through the gaze of the Other: "For the first time, the seeing that I am is for me really visible; for the first time I appear to myself completely turned inside out under my own eyes" (*VI,* 143).

The nature of body and world alike cannot be fully understood without reference to one final chiasmatic relation: that between the "visible and the invisible." Being is fleshed out by virtue of invisible dimensions that are *not* "non-visibles" opposed to perception but installed within the visible world (*VI,* 149, 215, 227–28, 236). For example, there is an invisibility that adheres to the perceiver. I never quite see another's perceptual powers and subjectivity when I gaze upon the object body. The seer is always *"a little behind," "a little further"* than the body I see (*VI,* 261). Correlatively, there is an invisible ideality that adheres to all sensible objects. The experienced world is not a collection of sense data but organized into meaningful gestalts. The visible profile of an object suggests its other hidden sides without which it would have no depth or solidity. In a sequence of musical notes I grasp a structure, an idea that resides in these sounds while never quite being reducible to them. This ideality of perception can emigrate "into another less heavy, more transparent body" (*VI,* 153), that of language. Yet even this "purified" ideality remains of the flesh. As I will later discuss, language always remains embodied in the signifier and the acts of reading and writing, speaking and listening. And while supplementing the sense of the perceptual world, words are always dependent upon it, drawing their meaning from an ideality that "already streams forth along the articulations of the esthesiological body, along the contours of the sensible things" (*VI,* 152).

This is but a brief description of Merleau-Ponty's richly textured notion of flesh, left uncompleted at his death. Yet it will suffice for the point I wish to make. All of the chiasmatic relations to which Merleau-Ponty refers are those involving the surface, ecstatic body. His philosophical language changes dramatically from his earlier *Phenomenology of Perception.* Yet the notion of flesh remains, in the broadest sense, an ontologizing of perception. It includes the intertwining of perceiver and perceived, the synergic crossing of different perceptual modalities, the reversibility of my perception with that of another, the fleshing out of perception with ideality and language. Another name Merleau-Ponty offers for the flesh is "Visibility" (*VI,* 139). It is the body surface, visioning and visible, that is taken as the *"exemplar sensible"* of flesh.

Viscerality

Yet this is not the body as a whole. We have seen that the perceptual and expressive surface always rests upon a hidden base. My inner organs are for the most part neither the agents nor objects of sensibility. They constitute their own circuitry of vibrant, pulsing life, which precedes the perceptual in fetal life, outruns it in sleep, sustains it from beneath at all moments. Rather than "Visibility," one might call this the dimension of "Viscerality." Like the Visible, the Visceral cannot be properly said to belong to the subject; it is a power that traverses me, granting me life in ways I have never fully willed nor comprehended.

This visceral circuit is intertwined, an identity-in-difference with the visible body. As has been shown, the two corporeal levels remain phenomenologically distinct. Yet I know that my visceral organs, my sleeping and fetal body, though ordinarily out of sight, are ultimately installed within the Visible. I can imagine the red, textured spectacle that awaits the surgeon who opens me up. Conversely, my powers of vision are installed in Viscerality, shaped and sustained by anonymous life. The eye lives only by virtue of the stomach's labor, and our digestive states help determine the quality and objects of our gaze.

This does not undermine but adds further dimension to Merleau-Ponty's chiasmatic analysis. The body is not just a chiasm of perceiver and perceived. Nor is it just an intertwining of perceptual powers, a "lateral, transversal" synergy of hands and eyes. There is also what one might call a "vertical" synergy; my surface powers rely upon deeper vegetative processes, as well as an unconscious fetal history and periods of sleep. More than just a "cluster of 'consciousnesses,' " my body is a chiasm of conscious and unconscious levels, a viscero-esthesiological being.

Flesh and Blood

While not fully captured in Merleau-Ponty's articulation of "flesh," this term could be expanded to include my findings. No quarrel is raised with the Merleau-Pontian emphasis on corporeality or his characterization of this as a chiasmatic series. But in order to emphasize the important supplementation the visceral chiasm effects, I will supplement Merleau-Ponty's language. Rather than using the term *flesh,* I will speak of the *flesh and blood.*

The very word *flesh* commonly refers to the body surface. (While this is true as well of the French original, *la chair,* this connotation is even more pronounced in the English translation.) Most typically, the flesh of an animal is equated with its superficial muscle and fatty tissue. One dictionary definition is simply "the surface of the human body, esp. with regard to its outward appearance."[51] The term thus already suggests the Merleau-Pontian tendency to focus on the sensorimotor surface of the body. Admittedly, *flesh,* as in the biblical sense, can also have a much broader significance, referring to the entire body or physical nature in general. Yet this ambiguous equation of the body-entire with the body-surface embodied in the very word *flesh* is precisely what I would wish to avoid.

The term *flesh and blood* suggests a dimension of depth hitherto unspoken. (Its nearest French equivalent is *en chair et en os*—"in flesh and bone.") Beneath the surface flesh, visible and tangible, lies a hidden vitality that courses within me. *Blood* is my metaphoric term for this viscerality. "Flesh and blood" expresses well the chiasmatic identity-in-difference of perceptual and visceral life. The expression itself appears in certain dictionaries as if one word. To be "flesh and blood" is clearly to be one thing, a life entire unto itself. Yet the "and" is never expunged, suggesting an *écart,* a divergence of two existential levels.[52*]

BODY AND WORLD

If the body is an *exemplar sensible,* the notion of flesh and blood must characterize not only the body in isolation but the relationship between body and world. In the perceptual chiasm, body and world reach out to each other from across an ineradicable space. Merleau-Ponty writes of a "thickness of flesh between the seer and the thing," a distance that is consonant with proximity (*VI,* 135). Perception is only possible via the mutual exteriority of perceiver and perceived.

Yet in addition to this perceptual communion of the flesh, I am sustained through a deeper "blood" relation with world. It is installed within me, not just encountered from without. The inanimate, calcified world supports my flesh from within in the form of bones. A world of organic, autonomous powers circulates within my visceral depths. Science tells me that some ten quadrillion bacteria live within my body. I cannot even claim my own cells fully as my own. In all probability, they evolved out of symbiotic relations between different prokaryotic cells, one living inside another.[53] My body everywhere bears the imprint of Otherness.

This encroachment of the world is renewed at every moment by visceral exchanges with the environment. In sleep I give myself over to anonymous breathing, relinquishing the separative nature of distance perception.[54] Even waking perception is ultimately in service to the visceral. In the most basic sense, the animal looks around to find things to eat and avoid being eaten.[55] (Merleau-Ponty's own term suggests this significance; *la chair* in French, like the English word, "flesh," commonly refers to meat, that which one devours.)[56*] As I eat, the thickness of the flesh that separates self from world melts away. No longer perceived across a distance, the world dissolves into my own blood, sustaining me from within via its nutritive powers. I am not just a gazing upon the world but one who feeds on it, drinks of it, breathes it in.

My relation to other subjects is, as well, a relation of flesh *and blood*. In Merleau-Ponty's description, I discover my own visibility and that of the world only fully through the gaze of another. Yet prior to this intertwining from without by two perceivers was an intertwining from within. As discussed, my lived body was formed from within that of another. I arose out of Viscerality, hidden from the gaze of my mother and preceding the birth of my own vision.[57]* Even my genes came not from perceptual but visceral chiasm. In the sexual act, my parents' bodies and cells intertwined, an identity-in-difference giving rise to me. My embryonic and fetal development then proceeded through a series of visceral *écarts:* the mitosis of my cells differentiating one from another, then giving rise to discrete but interrelated organ systems. The maternal/fetal relation is another chiasmatic identity-in-difference. While separate, we are enfolded together, sharing one pulsing bloodstream. Even after birth, through the act of breast-feeding, one body is nourished directly from the visceral production of the other.

Thus there is an intercorporeity of the blood of which the fleshly, perceptual encounter is a sublimated reflection. Though my own gestation is hidden, lost in depth disappearance, this bodily intertwining is never fully effaced from adult life. It is recapitulated in a limited way via the sexual act. It is experienced by women during pregnancy.[58]* It is sensed in the similarity of features my body shares with those of my parents. I am "of their flesh and blood," their genes residing within me. The visible image of our interpenetration is sketched right onto my face.

VISIBILITY AND INVISIBILITY

The final chiasm to which Merleau-Ponty refers is that of the visible and the invisible. This too demands re-vision. The invisibilities to which Merleau-Ponty refers all belong to the ecstatic body. I discussed in chapter 1 the invisibility of the perceiver, never quite coinciding with his or her visible organs. The invisibility of perceptual meaning as taken up into language will be discussed in chapter 4. Merleau-Ponty refers to these as "depths," giving dimension to the visible world (*VI,* 136, 149, 219, 236). Yet they always remain depths of a surface, adhering to the esthesiological and expressive body.

In this chapter, another sort of depth, invisibility, has been encountered. This is an invisible not just of the flesh, the perceptual circuit, but of the blood. The visceral organs, the fetal body from which I emerge, the sleeping body into which I lapse, are regions ineluctably hidden from perception. The life-world is textured by this unconscious vitality

as much as by the sublimations of language and thought. I have termed
this visceral invisible a depth disappearance, and the bulk of this chapter has been devoted to its expression.

A recognition of the visceral thus leads to a revision of all the chiasmatic
relations contained within the notion of flesh. The relations holding
within my own body, between body and world, self and Other, the visible and the invisible, attain their full depths only when this vital dimension is recalled. In each case a perceptual chiasm is supplemented by a
chiasm with, or of, the visceral. I am not merely consciousness, as Merleau-Ponty argues, but neither am I merely flesh. I am flesh and blood.

   To say I am flesh and blood—ecstatic and recessive being—is to radically revise our operative concept of self. To identify the self to any
extent with the body is considered in many spiritual traditions to be a
primary cause of suffering and separation. It is claimed that insofar as
we see ourselves as this located, material thing we deny our true identity
with the All. However, this separative stance may be a function not of
embodiment per se but of a restricted way of conceiving and living out
the body. For realized as flesh and blood, the lived body profoundly
challenges the separative stance. (I will explore this at greater length in
my closing chapter.) There is a Buddhist myth wherein the god Indra
has a net decorated with a bright jewel on each knot of the mesh. Each
jewel thus reflects all the other jewels unto infinity.[59] Reminiscent of the
philosophies of Leibniz or Whitehead, this myth suggests the mutual
mirroring of all points in the universe. Yet the lived body is just such a
jewel; my ecstatic flesh opens onto, mirrors the surrounding world of
other bodies. I am not then simply an "I" but all that I am not, a perspective upon the universe as a whole. Similarly, as "blood," or recessive
being, I find a consanguinity with processes that far outrun the traditional boundaries of self. It is not "I" as conscious, limited thing, that
first gave rise to or sustain my self, but a wider context of natural powers
of which I am but a partial expression. Each breath speaks of my depen-
dency upon the whole. As such, the universal or the "spiritual" need not
be conceived as something opposed to the flesh and blood. The body
itself proclaims spirit in our lives, that is, transcendence, mystery, and
interconnection.

3

The Dys-appearing Body

We are not tormented by some foreign agent, it is not an incident, a word, a thought, or even sickness or death, however we may acknowledge the powers of these: it is our own body. My own hand, my head, hurts me. The organs of the body, the heart, kidneys, stomach, function in a manner which is hidden and unconscious as far as I am concerned: now they refuse to serve, they are in revolt against me: they torment and rob me of my power over myself. This senseless abandonment of the human being to pain has its direct result in a cleavage of the self and the body.

Buytendijk, *Pain: Its Modes and Functions*

In previous chapters I have focused upon the body's tendency to disappear from awareness and action. This has proved to be a multidimensional phenomenon. As ecstatic, the body projects outside itself into the world. As recessive, the body falls back from its own conscious perception and control. In addition, the body simply "moves off to the side"; at any time, parts of the surface body are left unused or rendered subsidiary, placed in a background disappearance.

This provides us with a phenomenological resolution of the question with which we began this work: why, if human experience is rooted in the bodily, is the body so often absent from experience? I have attempted to show that certain modes of disappearance are essential to the body's functioning. As ecstatic/recessive being-in-the-world, the lived body is necessarily self-effacing.

Moreover, these modes of disappearance will help account for our cultural understanding of embodiment. In the West there has been a tendency to identify the essential self with the incorporeal mind, the body relegated to an oppositional moment. A phenomenological treatment of embodiment must not merely refute this view but account for its abiding power. I will suggest later that it is *the body's own tendency toward self-concealment* that allows for the possibility of its neglect or deprecation. Our organic basis can be easily forgotten due to the reticence of visceral processes. Intentionality can be attributed to a disembodied mind, given the self-effacement of the ecstatic body. As these disappearances particularly characterize normal and healthy functioning, forgetting about or "freeing oneself" from the body takes on a positive valuation. The import of such life-world experiences in determining metaphysical and ethical attitudes toward the body will be taken up in part 2 of this work.

However, before this is possible I must continue the phenomenological exploration, albeit with a twist. I have been discussing the body as "absent," etymologically "to be away." The ecstatic-recessive awayness of the body accounts for its withdrawal from experience. However, the character of "being away" is also an ingredient in many experiences we do have of our own bodies. My own body may feel away from me, something problematic and foreign, even at moments of its most intimate disclosure. The "absence" of the body, in a primordial sense, infects its presence from the very start. In this chapter I will focus on those phenomena in which the body manifests as a problematic or disharmonious thing, and is therefore experienced as a "being-away."

This is not meant to suggest that such is the invariant essence of corporeal experience. I do not intend a general survey of the various modes of apprehending one's body: its kinesthesias and coenesthesias, pleasures as well as pains, visual and tactile apprehensions, both direct and mediated through mirrorings, all of these supplemented and interpreted through the gaze and response of others, the vagaries of our psychological history, the scientific knowledge current in our time. The weaving of a body-image out of such diverse threads is an ongoing matter of study for psychologists and philosophers alike. However, such will not form the subject of this chapter.

For several reasons, I am analyzing only a particular class of body experiences, those involving problematic or dysfunctional relations. First, as previously mentioned, this will further my discussion of the "absence" or "awayness" of the body which, to be fully grasped, must be seen as ingredient within modes of self-presence. Second, such disruptive experiences have, as I will later argue, a certain phenomenological power and demand quality that make them central in shaping our views on embodiment. Finally, for this reason, such experiences are important vis-à-vis the history of the concept of the body. Insofar as the body seizes our awareness particularly at times of disturbance, it can come to appear "Other" and opposed to the self. Such experiences then play a part in buttressing Cartesian dualism.

Pain

In discussing the problematic presencing of the body I will start with the example of physical pain. Even in this seemingly simple sensation there is the seed of a body-self division. I will then expand discussion to the broader context in which pain is often situated: that of disease and dysfunction. As in the previous chapters, a phenomenological example will provide the point of entry.

A man is playing tennis. His attention dwells upon the ball flying toward him, the movements of his opponent, the corner of the court toward which he aims his return. He is already flexing in preparation for this shot and a subsequent charge to net. The closer the ball approaches, the more it acts to focus his attention and posture until at the exactly right moment, without the need of explicit thought or will, his body uncoils to meet it with force.

But as he swings he feels a sudden pain in the chest. His attention now shifts to the expanding focus of pain. The concerns with the game that a moment before were paramount—the perceptions of the ball, the court, the tricky wind, the attempt to intuit and outwit his opponent—all this recedes before the insistent ache. He raises and lowers his arms to see if the pain is muscular in origin, and flexes his torso in an attempt to reduce discomfort. But the pain hangs on, centered in the chest and spreading up the shoulder. He is distressed and a little fearful. He stops the game which, in an experiential sense, is already something far away.

Prior to the onset of pain, the body of the tennis player stands in the threefold disappearance previously described. Attention is ecstatically distributed to distant points. Parts of the body are backgrounded and forgotten as all power centers in the swing. A metabolic machinery supplies the player with energy, without demanding his attention or guidance. The game is made possible only by this bodily self-concealment.

Yet this structure is lacerated by a single moment of pain. The player is called back from ecstatic engagement to a focus upon the state of his own body. A background region, the chest, is now thematized. Assuming for the moment the pain is cardiac in origin, a once tacit viscerality now floods through perception and cries out for action. Pain can thus overcome focal, background, and depth disappearance alike. How does pain bring about this transformation? The answer, though seemingly quite obvious, is only unfolded by a detailed analysis.

First, and most basically, pain effects what I will term a *sensory intensification*. A region of the body that may have previously given forth little in the way of sensory stimuli suddenly speaks up. As discussed in the last chapter, this is typical of the inner body, often silent except at times of discomfort. Even body regions that are ordinarily perceptible still present a heightened call when in pain. The chest of the tennis player was already a place of heavy breathing, the smell and dampness of sweat, wind against the skin. Yet these stimuli are surpassed and overwhelmed by the pain. The body is so constructed with its abundant number, variety, and distribution of pain receptors that this sensation is one of the most intense we experience. Indeed it is characteristic of other sensory possibilities to turn into pain when their levels become too great: the light too bright or the sound too loud, the water too hot or cold, the annoying tickle that reaches unsupportable levels.

Pain asserts itself not only via its sensory intensification but through its characteristic temporality: that which I will term its *episodic structure*. We usually notice in the ongoing stream of sensation that which stands out as episodic and discrete. This is frequently the case with pain. It is not a constant accompaniment of normal bodily activity but tends to arise at times of unusual stress or trauma. The feeling of the wind and sweat on the tennis player's chest, the effort of breathing, the kinesthesias of muscles and joints, were for him continual, if modulating, stimuli. As such they could sink to an unthematized background. By contrast, the pain arises suddenly. It punctures the scene with novelty. Even pains of a more chronic nature are often marked with an episodic nature, changing in their character and intensity according to one's activity, position, or visceral periodicities. Feelings of general neutrality or well-being are typically amorphous, marked neither by definable beginnings and ends nor abrupt transformations. Pain, as a symptom of the problematic, frequently is.

Even relatively constant pains participate in this episodic temporality via their continual reassertion of presence. It is characteristic of most stimuli to experientially recede as they persist over time. We notice the noise when the air conditioning is first turned on but soon forget it. When we touch something, there is an initial feeling of pressure that gradually fades until the point of contact becomes more difficult to feel. There are a variety of neurological correlates to such experiential extinguishings. On the peripheral level, most sensory receptors have mechanisms for either partial or complete "adaptation" to repetitive stimuli. Over time, as a result of mechanical or chemical adjustments, receptors simply cease firing or decrease their rate of response to the same stimulus. Pain receptors, on the other hand, adapt either little or not at all. They react strongly as long as the pain stimulus continues, some even increasing in sensitivity over time.[1] Biologically this has a clear usefulness. The animal is propelled to attend and act however long the damaging stimulus persists. Experientially, though, this can be most annoying. A chronic pain for which one has no solution continues to grab the attention with undiminished intensity. To an extent, one can accept or become accustomed to such pain. But it still retains something of an episodic character. It is as if the pain were ever born anew, although nothing whatsoever has changed.

In addition to such features of intensity and temporality, pain has a unique qualitative feel that sets it off from other sensory experiences: namely, it *hurts*. Pain is the very concretization of the unpleasant, the aversive. It places upon the sufferer what I will term an *affective call*. One's attention is summoned by the gnawing, distasteful quality of pain in a way that it would not be by a more neutral stimulus. The feelings of wind, sweat, breath, and effort placed no great affective demand on the tennis player. His attention was free to roam elsewhere despite strong bodily sensations. However, when the character of these changed from those of vigorous well-being to the unpleasant, it is as if a magnet had reversed poles, reorganizing the experiential field inward.

This affective call has a quality of compulsion. I am seized by the pain in a way I am not by other experiences of the body. I can choose to look in the mirror or not, to pay attention or not to my kinesthesias. Even strong pleasures, such as those of a sexual nature, may leave one's thoughts wandering. Aesthetic, objective, or pleasurable self-encounters retain a large volitional element. With pain this is less the case, not only because of its typically involuntary etiology but because of the quality of the sensation itself. The tennis player did not choose to stop his game and focus upon his chest. He is seized by a power holding sway over him. In the face of pain, one's whole being is forcibly reoriented.

This is not to say that the call of pain is irresistible. The tennis player, if in the midst of a crucial point, might have kept his concentration upon the game. A trained yogi can learn to ignore pain entirely and suppress reflexive motor responses. But the powerful distractions, training, or acts of will necessary to resist pain's call bear testimony to its original strength.

I have briefly characterized pain qua sensory mode. The sensory intensification it brings into play, combined with an episodic temporality and affective call establishes its peculiar hold upon our attention. Yet pain, like any other experiential mode, cannot be reduced to a set of immediate sensory qualities. It is ultimately a manner of being-in-the-world. As such, pain reorganizes our lived space and time, our relations with others and with ourselves. The full phenomenological import of pain is only revealed when set within this broader context. Here pain effects what I will term an *intentional disruption* and a *spatiotemporal constriction*. Correlatively, the painful body emerges as an *alien presence* that exerts upon us a *telic demand*.

I will begin by examining the *intentional disruption* that accompanies pain. Prior to the onset of pain, the lived body of the tennis player is an openness upon the world. It is a center from which the rays of intentionality radiate outward. The player is ecstatically *with* the ball, the distant side of the court, the projected responses of his opponent. To use Polanyi's language, he lives from his body to the world. It is this relation in all its dimensions that is disrupted by the call of pain. No longer simply a "from" structure, the painful body becomes that *to* which he attends. As the body surfaces thematically its transitive use is disrupted. That is, the game comes to a stop. First, the tennis player may be unable to focus perceptually on the game as his chest throbs. Second, the severe demand of the pain can serve to immobilize him—we thus speak of being "frozen in agony." Third, even if he could resume the game, he might not risk it; movement could aggravate the pain or the injury that caused it. Finally, he may simply lose interest in the game. The highly affective and significant call of pain renders unimportant projects that previously seemed crucial.[2]

As the world of the game is disrupted, so is the connection with another. A moment before the two players were bound together. They shared the court, the flight of the ball, the wind, the joy of effort and competition. Their thoughts intertwined around the goal of victory, the mutual anticipation of each other's strategy. But pain strikes one alone. Unlike the feel of the cool wind, pain is marked by an interiority that another cannot share. As Scarry notes, pain "achieves it aversiveness in part by bringing about, even within the radius of several feet, this absolute split between one's sense of one's own reality and the reality of other persons."[3] The person in pain may reach out more to others, yet this is in response to the individualizing effects of suffering. As Updike writes:

> [Pain] shows us, too, how those around us
> do not, and cannot, share
> our being; though men talk animatedly
> and challenge silence with laughter
>
> and women bring their engendering smiles
> and eyes of famous mercy,
> these kind things slide away
> like rain beating on a filthy window
>
> when pain interposes.[4]

Such is not the case with pleasure. While sensations of pleasure and well-being may call one back to one's body, there is rarely the same character of disrupted intentionality vis-à-vis objects or other people. Pleasures are usually secured through the body's commerce with the world effecting a satisfaction of need or desire. Moreover, such pleasurable sensations are primarily experienced as in and from the world, not merely my own body. I find myself enjoying the taste *of the food,* not that of my own taste buds. Pain, on the other hand, is usually experienced as located within the confines of my flesh. A general indicator of tissue damage, its sensory character may be quite independent of, and persist in the absence of, its environmental cause.[5]

Pleasures, as more tied to a common world, also tend to maintain our intentional links with other people. We feast and drink with friends, making of our enjoyment a common bond. It is our means of connection, not, as Updike writes of pain, a "filthy window" interposed between us. The primal image of pleasure, that of the infant feeding, depends upon a caretaker's presence. In adulthood, many pleasures, such as the sexual, are still secured primarily with and through others. The feel, the look, the invitation, of the desired one is precisely what arouses one's own bodily response. Even solitary sexuality is usually motivated by another's body as pictured or imagined.

Thus, as Buytendijk discusses, pleasure and the happiness with which it is often accompanied is naturally "expansive."[6] We fill our bodies with what they lack, open up to the stream of the world, reach out to others. In contrast, pain tends to induce self-reflection and isolation. It effects a *spatiotemporal constriction.*

The tendency of pain to disrupt our intentionalities never leads to a complete collapse of the world. It is our nature, as being-in-the-world, to inhabit a significant continuum of space and time, projects and goals. However, the new world into which we are thrust by pain has a constricted aspect. The expanse of the distance senses is replaced by the oppressive nearness of coenesthesia. We are no longer dispersed out *there* in the world, but suddenly congeal right *here.* Our attention is drawn back not only to our own bodies but often to a particular body part. In Scarry's words, intense pain is "experienced spatially as either the contraction of the universe down to the immediate vicinity of the body or as the body swelling to fill the entire universe."[7]

A motoric constriction accompanies the perceptual. As discussed, pain and the disability it signals often restrict our possibilities of movement. Things we once could do now seem impossible or uninteresting. Even if we can move, we often find it useless. The tennis player tests out different positions and motions but none relieve his pain. With chronic suffering there is nowhere to go, nothing to do, no escape. Space loses its normal directionality as the world ceases to be the locus of purposeful action.

Physical suffering constricts not only the spatial but the temporal sphere. As it pulls us back to the *here,* so severe pain summons us to the *now.* Prior to injury, the tennis player roamed the future, already preparing for the next shot and seeking a desired victory. Pain seizes him back to the present. Its intensity and affectivity demand his attention right now.

This temporal constriction is characteristic of chronic pain as well. While the body in well-being can explore the far reaches of time through memory and imagination, such possibilities constrict when we are in pain. With chronic suffering a painless past is all but forgotten. While knowing intellectually that we were once not in pain we have lost the bodily memory of how this felt. Similarly, a painless future may be unimaginable. In the words of Emily Dickinson:

> Pain—has an Element of Blank—
> It cannot recollect
> When it began—or if there were
> A time when it was not—
>
> It has no Future—but itself—
> Its Infinite contain
> Its Past—enlightened to perceive
> New Periods—of Pain.[8]

Thus, pain exerts a phenomenologically "centripetal" force, gathering space and time inward to the center. We are ceaselessly reminded of the here-and-now body. The very aversiveness of pain may also lead to a counteraction; I discuss elsewhere a "centrifugal" movement in which we seek to escape this hold of pain by focusing outward upon the world, or dwelling in our past or a hoped-for future.[9] Yet even such a movement outwards bears witness to the original constrictiveness of pain. The body is no longer a nullpoint but an active presence whose call we must resist.

The disruption and constriction of one's habitual world thus correlates with a new relation to one's body. In pain, the body or a certain part of the body emerges as an *alien presence*.[10] The sensory insistence of pain draws the corporeal out of self-concealment, rendering it thematic. No event more radically and inescapably reminds us of our bodily presence.[11] Yet at the same time pain effects a certain alienation. White and Sweet report that their patients almost universally describe their pain as an "it," separate from the "I."[12] The painful body is often experienced as something foreign to the self.

There are several reasons for this. Most basically, this combination of identity and difference pervades all of perception. To return to Merleau-Pontian language, the perceptual bond is always based on the *écart* (divergence). To perceive anything is both to enter into a communality with it and to confront it as something that is at least marginally separate from the perceiver. Whenever our body becomes an object of perception, even though it perceives itself, an element of distance is introduced. I no longer simply "am" my body, the set of unthematized powers from which I exist. Now I "have" a body, a perceived object in the world.

However, this *écart* of the flesh does not account for the distinctiveness of pain. Pain engenders a further dimension of alienation that is not a part of neutral or pleasurable self-experience. There are admittedly certain pains, such as that of the athlete pressing against limits, that are congruent with life projects and have a positive significance. ("No pain, no gain.") Yet this is the exception rather than the rule. In most cases pain is an unwanted and aversive phenomenon that forces itself upon us against our will. Moreover, it threatens the very routines and goals by which we define our identity. Aversive, involuntary, and disruptive, the painful body emerges as a foreign thing.[13]

This cleavage between body and self is not only initiated by the pain but may also serve as an adaptive response to it. As Bakan points out, when the affected part of the body becomes "other" to the ego, one becomes more ready to take whatever means are necessary to rid oneself of it.[14] A tooth may need to be pulled or a limb amputated; one is prepared for physical invasions and separations by an existential separation already effected. With pain that cannot be so removed, a process of distancing still provides consolation. To experience the painful body as merely an "it," that which is separate from the essential self, yields some relief and reestablishes one's integrity in the face of an overwhelming threat.

Thus, the sense of the body as an alien thing does not arise solely in the objectifications of the modern physician.[15] Prior to visiting the doctor's office, the pain and disability of the patient have already laid the groundwork for a distanced perspective. Plügge, the German physician and philosopher, has discussed this phenomenon eloquently. He argues that the sheer "thinglike" nature of the body, as reified in Cartesian metaphysics, first surfaces in life-world experiences of effort, fatigue, disease, and the like.[16]

To fully understand the alien presence of the painful body it is necessary to look at the projects it brings into play. Pain exerts a *telic demand* upon us. While calling us to the now, its distasteful quality also establishes a futural goal: to be free of pain. As Sartre writes, "pain-consciousness is a project toward a further consciousness which would be empty of all pain; that is, to a consciousness whose contexture, whose being-there would be not painful."[17] The sensory aversiveness and world disruptions effected by pain cry out for removal. This goal is built into our body's neuromuscular circuitry; we reflexively withdraw from a pain stimulus. On a more complex level, pain's telic demand includes what I will term a *hermeneutical* and a *pragmatic* moment.

In the hermeneutical moment, suffering gives rise to a search for interpretation and understanding.[18] The tennis player stops the game not simply out of an inability but also in a positive quest for meaning. He wants to know about the origin, extent, and significance of the pain. Only then will he be in a position to take reparatory action or cope with the pain's existential challenge. As Bakan writes:

> To attempt to understand the nature of pain, to seek to find its meaning, is already to respond to an imperative of pain itself. No experience demands and insists upon interpretation in the same way. Pain forces the question of its meaning, and especially of its cause, insofar as cause is an important part of its meaning. In those instances in which pain is intense and intractable and in which its causes are obscure, its demand for interpretation is most naked, manifested in the sufferer asking "Why?" Thus, our very effort to understand the nature of pain is natural, much as it is natural for man to concern himself with disease.[19]

When in pain, the body becomes the object of an ongoing interpretive quest. We obsessively probe and palpate even when this increases discomfort. We read books on the body, seeking self-diagnosis, or ask friends for answers. We go back through the past, reflecting on our bodily history and possible origins of the current problem. We pose tests to see what diminishes or increases pain. Even at times when the discomfort disappears we wonder why and hold watchful vigil. If we finally seek out a healthcare provider, this is hardly an abandonment of self-exploration. Rather, the treater's gaze provides an extension of our own. Through the mediation of another, we come to see our body in a series of technologically and conceptually extended ways that otherwise would be unavailable.

Sensations of well-being rarely induce such corporeal hermeneutics. One may savor particular pleasures, but they do not demand continued self-reflection or the use of diagnostic specialists. In pleasure there is ordinarily no threat to one's being, no mysterious etiology, no aversiveness to be removed. As such one simply "enjoys" the pleasure. Szasz writes:

> *Whereas "pain" is a command for action, "pleasure"* (which may be equated here with contentment or happiness) *calls for no action.* The ego's essential experience and wish is for *no change* from the existing situation.[20]

The aversiveness of pain does call for change. Hence, the hermeneutical moment is ultimately involved with a pragmatic goal: getting rid of, or mastering, suffering.[21]* My own body becomes the object not just of perception and interpretation but of action. I seek medication, physical therapies, whatever will help. My projects are reorganized around the attempt to cope with or remove the pain. Instead of just acting *from* the body, I act *toward* it. This goal of pain removal is but one of many valued ends and may at times be overridden. One may even consciously stimulate pain, as in forms of religious asceticism or puberty rites. However, the power of such practices to test the will originates in pain's telic demand. One must exercise strength of character to overcome the powerful urge to escape.

Disease

I have analyzed the ways in which the painful body emerges from disappearance to become a thematic object. Pain exerts a power that reverberates throughout the phenomenological field, shifting our relations both to the world and to ourselves. There is a disruption of intentional linkages and a constriction of our spatiality and temporality to their embodied center. The painful body emerges as alien presence, its telic demand reorganizing around it ongoing projects of interpretation and repair.

Immediate sensation can thus inaugurate a bodily appearance. If the pain is transitory and of no great consequence one may within minutes return to one's habitual world. However, such phenomenological shifts can be of a more enduring nature, stretching over days, months, or years and resulting from long-standing physical processes. This is often the case in situations of disease.

To explore this phenomenon is on the one hand simply to broaden the context of our previous discussion. Pain is a common accompaniment of disease to the point where the distinction between the two blur. However, they are hardly identical. There are many pains unconnected to a disease state. I may, for example, induce discomfort by pinching myself or enduring a long-distance run. Conversely, there are many disease processes (e.g., dermatological) that are painless. Other diseases give rise to pain and discomfort only on a sporadic basis. The common tendency to associate pain and disease is not explained simply on the basis of their frequent physical contiguity. It rests, as well, upon a phenomenological association: disease tends to effect many of the same experiential shifts as does pain.

In illustrating this point, I will not attempt a detailed phenomenology of disease states. There are several excellent examples in the literature.[22] Nor will I seek the elusive definition of *disease* versus *health*[23] or systematically contrast, as some authors have, "disease" as a scientifically interpreted physiological event with the "illness" actually experienced by the sufferer.[24] The very term *disease* (dis-ease) expresses well the experienced loss of comfort and possibility that often accompanies physiological disruption.

To orient the discussion, I will continue my previous example to its morbid conclusion.

After his pain fails to subside, the tennis player pays a visit to the hospital, learning to his dismay that he has had a heart attack of moderate severity. For several days he is confined to a hospital bed, his movement severely restricted. He is permitted to increase his activity upon returning home, but only gradually. A continued sense of limits remain with him; many things he once did he no longer dares risk, or at least not without some planning and trepidation. His attention often returns to his chest as he watches for the least sign of pain or irregularity. There is an expectant distrust, a subliminal awareness of the heart that never fully disappears even when his pain has long been absent. He resumes playing tennis but now as much for the sake of rebuilding the heart as for enjoyment.

Finally, the day comes when there is a second heart attack more disabling than the first. A weak heart now places severe limits on our subject's activity; he experiences a generalized heaviness and fatigue and cannot walk far because of shortness of breath. Sometimes a difficulty with breathing wakes him in the middle of the night. Diuretics and other medications lessen some of the symptoms but are in no way curative. His appetite decreases for food, and for life in general. The everyday concerns of others recede as he finds himself thinking more frequently about death.

Buytendijk writes, "being ill is before all alienation from the world."[25] As the above example suggests, disease, like pain, effects a disruption of intentional links and a spatiotemporal constriction. This may first originate in the immediate call of pain and discomfort. However, it is hardly confined to this. Long after the pain of the first heart attack had passed, the disruption of the tennis player's world remains. Confined to a hospital bed during the period of recovery, he is removed from the meaningful context of job, home, friends, and family. Even frequent visitors cannot know or share fully the experience he has been through. Spatiality and temporality constrict to the world of the hospital, the slow progress of recovery. As van den Berg describes, the sick person may hear the sounds of the street from the window as others go about their business.

However, this world, which the patient had until recently inhabited, now echoes as though from an inaccessible distance.[26]

After the first heart attack, a period of withdrawal is enforced by doctor's orders. The patient must rest in order to avoid exacerbating the infarct. Hence, part of the disruption and constrictiveness of illness is often reflectively willed as a therapeutic mode. However, the disease itself inaugurates a constriction that does not end with the period of formal confinement. Plügge describes how cardiac patients, as exemplified by the above subject, experience a reduced sense of time and space.[27] After a heart attack, such patients no longer want to look into the distant future. A landscape is viewed not as a field of possibility but of difficulties to negotiate. The ordinary sense of free and spontaneous movement is now replaced by calculated effort; one does not want to take chances. Etymologically, "ease" comes from the French word *aise,* originally meaning "elbow room" or "opportunity." This experience of world-as-opportunity is precisely what dis-ease calls into question.

This is even more the case when serious illness radically truncates our physical capabilities. After the second heart attack our subject is simply unable to do many things he previously could. A diffuse weakness and exhaustion make vigorous movement impossible. In addition to imposing such generalized constrictions, each specific disease is characterized by its idiosyncratic motifs of disruption. For example, because of the collection of fluid in the lungs, cardiac failure may prohibit particular sleeping postures.

Hence, disease, even more than pain, is typified by complex patterns of dysfunction. The "I can" of bodily ecstasis is disturbed. What results is not, however, identical to the "I cannot" of the recessive body. The latter refers to the fact that one's visceral functions continually and necessarily elude direct control. One is simply *un-able.* In disease, one is actively *dis-abled.* Abilities that were previously in one's command and rightfully belong to the habitual body have now been lost. This could be termed the phenomenon of the "I no longer can."[28] When sick, I no longer can engage the world as once I could. There may be nostalgia for lost possibility, hope for its return, fear that disability will further spread.

As in the case of pain, this intentional disruption and spatiotemporal constriction correlates with a heightened thematization of the body. The diseased body introduces its own episodic temporality of rally and relapse, which makes it stand out from the amorphous time of health. A telic demand for interpretation and repair further turns the sick person's focus inward. The consequent self-preoccupation of the ill is a well-recognized phenomenon. The invalid's meticulous attention to the least bodily functions, the careful consideration of all acts as to their harmful or therapeutic effects, has both its tragic and comic aspects.

This alien presencing of the body in disease is a more complex matter than is the case with simple pain. We may first be seized by any of a variety of sensations. The body when ill is a concert master not only of pain but of warmth and cold, bloating, pressures, fatigues, nausea, tinglings, itches. Then again, our attention may be called not to changes in inner sensation but in outer appearance. A skin disease may simply look bad though no discomfort is experienced. Some syndromes are defined as diseases primarily because they are disfiguring or embarrassing, offending our sense of the proper body; Engelhardt terms this the aesthetic criterion of disease.[29] In such cases our body takes on an alien presence insofar as it is an object of pity or disgust. Its appearance no longer expresses one's own wishes and personality but the hegemony of an occupying force. In general, hospitalized patients are often highly aware not simply of the internal but the external body, with its sallow look, distasteful odor, and embarrassing excretory needs.

The general disability characteristic of sickness is also a factor in bodily thematization. Whereas one's attention is called to the body immediately in discomfort and disfigurement, this is not always the case with mild disability; secondary reflection may be necessary. Plügge describes how, given the ecstatic nature of embodiment, certain patients experience *Missbefinden* ("feeling poorly") as a change primarily in their outer world.[30] Habitual actions seem more difficult to do, and the environment takes on an unappetizing or resistant demeanor. This stage may continue for months or even years. However, for the most part, one is finally induced by such difficulties to reflect back upon the body itself. "Perhaps there is something wrong with me—perhaps I am sick—I should see a doctor."

If illness presents itself not as vague *Missbefinden* but as a sharp and specific curtailment of function, this surfacing of the body is more immediate. I know something is wrong with me when the morning comes and I cannot get out of bed. The tennis player in congestive heart failure is aware of the body in everything he cannot do. "It" is what stops him from going to the kitchen. "It" stands between him and all aspects of a normal life. The body can interfere in this way only because it is the power behind such acts, the locus of our sensorimotor abilities. When functioning well this body is a transparency through which we engage the world. As Plügge and Kohn write, well-being is "in general, synonymous with my noticing nothing about my body."[31] Yet when the body is rendered opaque through loss of function, we become aware of it as alien presence.

This principle comes sharply into play when we are threatened by death. Taken for granted as a ground of vitality, the body is often explicitly thematized when death approaches. With life-threatening illness, as in the case of the tennis player, not just this or that action, intentional link, or pleasurable sensation are undermined; everything at once comes under threat. Death suggests the "I no longer can" of all. As Heidegger points out, this dying is never simply a physical event, but of existential and ontological import.[32] Yet at the same time it *is* a physical event belonging to a bodily history I never fully intend. The illness progresses with its own characteristic course and temporality; the tennis player will see his grandchildren next Christmas *if* health permits. He is subject to what Ricoeur calls the "corporeal involuntary,"[33] a power, temporality, and set of demands with which the experienced "I" never quite coincides. Thus, Tolstoy describes Ivan Ilych contemplating his pain and approaching death:

> He would go to his study, lie down, and again be alone with *It:* face-to-face with *It.* And nothing could be done with *It* except to look at it and shudder.[34]

As the sensation of pain is the harbinger of illness, and as illness foretells the coming of death, so the alien presence of the body expands until it can threaten the entirety of one's world.

Dys-appearance

In order to understand the principle at play here, it is useful to refer back to Heidegger's discussion of the tool.[35] Heidegger notes that the "ready-to-hand" tool withdraws insofar as it functions unproblematically. We concern ourselves then with the work and its goals, the "towards-which" the tool is used. Only when the tool manifests a certain "un-readiness-to-hand" by virtue of becoming unuseable, missing, or standing in the way, must we take explicit account of it. It stands forth as "present-at-hand" because of a dysfunctional break in its employment.

As I discussed, the tool can best be understood as an "incorporated" structure. It withdraws insofar as it is brought within the tacit body. It might then be expected that the mode of presencing characteristic of the tool also derives from its bodily participation. This is confirmed by our previous examples. It is characteristic of the body itself to presence in times of breakdown or problematic performance. The tool, as an extended part of the body, merely participates in the same phenomenological structure. At moments of breakdown I experience *to* my body, not simply *from* it. My body demands a direct and focal thematization. In contrast to the "disappearances" that characterize ordinary functioning, I will term this the principle of *dys-appearance*. That is, the body *appears* as thematic focus, but precisely as in a *dys* state—*dys* is from the Greek prefix signifying "bad," "hard," or "ill," and is found in English words such as "dysfunctional." The full significance of the term *dys-appearance* will shortly be explored. Prior to that, I will further unfold the range of examples to which this principle can apply.

An exploration of pain and disease has provided an initial point of entry. These aversive states bring corporeality to explicit awareness for the sufferer. Indeed, the sick body partakes in all the modes of un-read-iness-to-hand that Heidegger describes in relation to the tool. At times of illness one may experience one's body as more or less "unuseable." It no longer can do what once it could. Certain possibilities of sensation and action, certain resources of energy, are simply "missing." The body that remains, as Heidegger writes of equipment, "reveals itself as something just present-at-hand and no more, which cannot be budged without the thing that is missing."[36] Finally, the sick body may be experienced as that which "stands in the way," an obstinate force interfering with our projects. As death approaches, these modes only heighten. The corpse is the very essence of the unuseable, that from which all life is missing, that which threatens to stand between us and the accomplishment of our ends.

Dys-appearance, however, is not confined to pathological or terminal states. When normal physiology reaches certain functional limits it seizes our attention. We remember the body at times of hunger, thirst, strong excretory needs, and the like. It is biologically adaptive that we recall our situation at such moments and that their unpleasantness exert a telic demand for removal. Cases of weakness, dizziness, or fatigue operate similarly. Plügge describes how in the initial stages of tiredness the environment itself seems to change, losing its variety and attractiveness. However, when this progresses to real exhaustion, one's focus is taken over by the body. One's limbs come to feel like heavy prostheses, as movements must be attended to and actively willed.[37]

Dys-appearance characterizes not only the limits of vital functioning but those of affectivity. I may become aware of a raging anger twisting my body or a lethargic depression leaving me limp. I feel these emotions holding sway within me as an alien presence that I cannot shake. Anxiety provides a good example of this phenomenon. Reading a paper at an important conference I discover my hands becoming clammy, my voice beginning to crack. My heart is racing and my breathing takes on a choked quality. Try as I might to focus on my talk, my attention is pulled back to these physical manifestations. I watch and try to control them, breathing deeply to calm myself and modulating my voice so that my nervousness will not show. This anxiety is undoubtedly mine, but is also something from without, fighting my efforts at mastery.

This affective disturbance not only gives rise to bodily self-consciousness but may originally have been the result of it. In this case, my anxiety was first stimulated by the hundreds of pairs of eyes focused upon me. My self-awareness in the face of this Gaze led to nervousness and consequent bodily symptoms. This illustrates a correlative principle to the one I have been exploring. In dys-appearance, the body is thematized at times of dysfunction or problematic operation. Conversely, thematizing the body can itself bring about dysfunction. For, as has been discussed, that from which we act or perceive necessarily operates in a tacit fashion. Insofar as we thematize the "from" term we tend to disrupt its ecstatic projectivity. Polanyi gives an example: "if a pianist shifts his attention from the piece he is playing to the observation of what he is doing with his fingers while playing it, he gets confused and may have to stop."[38] The principle of dys-appearance is thus potentially "bidirectional," dysfunction and body awareness engendering one another. This need not be the case, for self-awareness can allow us to seek help and effect repair. However, it can also exacerbate problems, intensifying anxiety or a slump in performance.

Bodily dys-appearance may be triggered not only by vital or affective disturbance but by dysfunction in the motor sphere. I forget my feet until the moment I stumble. A poor backhand makes a tennis player self-aware. When shot after shot goes into the net, I begin to reflect upon and adjust my swing. A heightened body awareness not only arises at such times when mastered skills go awry but also characterizes the initial acquisition of motor schemas. As discussed, when first learning a skill one needs to concentrate explicitly on its bodily performance though this will later become tacit. There is a dis-ease with the novel situation that provokes bodily dys-appearance.

Perceptual as well as motor difficulties may stimulate this self-consciousness. I am ordinarily oblivious to the act of sight until I see something that strikes me as impossible. Then I "rub my eyes," "pinch myself," that is, check my own perceptual conditions. When the world at large becomes strangely blurred I remember to go for an eye exam. As long as perception presents no problem my body disappears. But in situations of questionable or blocked perception, I am called to reflect back upon bodily states. These are the focus not only of attention but of action; I change my position, get a better angle, or supplement my perceptual possibilities in some way. As I will discuss in chapter 5, such examples of perceptual dys-appearance have a philosophical significance. That the body is remembered particularly at times of error and limitation helps to explain the Cartesian epistemological distrust of the body. Largely forgotten as a ground of knowledge, the body surfaces as the seat of deception.

I have surveyed a series of examples wherein the body presences as a result of disturbances in coenesthesia, health, homeostatic and vital functioning, affectivity, motility, and perception. These problematic situations initiate dys-appearance through a variety of mechanisms. Sensations of pain and discomfort exert an immediate call, based on the body's prereflective circuitry. On the other hand, self-awareness may result from secondary reflection, as in subtle *Missbefinden* or sensorimotor error. A disruption in world-relations leads one to reflect back upon one's bodily performance. In either case, the negativity of such disruptions further inaugurates a telic demand for repair. In order to return to normal mastery, the body itself becomes the focus of ongoing hermeneutic and pragmatic projects.

I have used the term "dys-appearance" to refer to this thematization of the body which accompanies dysfunction and problematic states. Dys-*appearance* is a mode, though by no means the only one, through which the body *appears* to explicit awareness. As such, it effects an attentional reversal of all the types of disappearance that I have heretofore explored. Thus, the two words, *dys-appearance* and *disappearance* have an antonymic significance. Yet at the same time, the homonymity of these words is meant to suggest the deep relation between these modes. It is precisely because the normal and healthy body largely disappears that direct experience of the body is skewed toward times of dysfunction. These phenomenological modes are mutually implicatory, as can be seen in relation both to the body surface and the visceral depths.

In the case of the body surface, we live from our organs ecstatically to the world; I have termed this *focal disappearance*. Self-forgetting is thus intrinsic to body function. Yet, it is also for this reason that self-presencing particularly arises at times when ecstasis is disturbed, as by disease or dysfunction. Attention must then be turned back upon the body. Disappearance and dys-appearance are thus implied correlatively by bodily ecstasis.

This correlativity holds true as well vis-à-vis the body's recessive aspect. My viscerality is constructed to proceed largely in silence without the knowledge or control of the conscious self. This is what I have termed *depth disappearance*. However, this is also why visceral awareness is most associated with modes of discomfort and illness. It is at such times, signaling tissue damage or disrupted homeostasis, that the intervention of the conscious "I" becomes a requirement.

In dys-appearance, the antonym/homonym of what was previously discussed, the prefix *dys* evokes several levels of meaning. As mentioned, *dys,* in Greek, signifies "bad," "hard," or "ill." (It is the opposite of *eu,* the prefix meaning "good" or "well.") As discussed, the body frequently appears at such times when it is ill, confronts the hard or problematic situation, or in some way performs badly. This Greek sense is preserved in English words such as "dysfunction," as well as in many terms for illnesses, such as "dysentery," "dyslexia," "dyskinesia," or "dysmenorrhea."

However, *dys* is also a variant spelling, now somewhat archaic, of the Latin root *dis.* This originally had the meaning of "away," "apart," or "asunder." I employ the spelling *dys* both for its Greek connotations and to allow for a visual mark of difference between "dys-appearance" and the modes of "disappearance" previously discussed. However, the Latin significance is also fully intended. The body in dys-appearance is marked by being away, apart, asunder. This is true along several dimensions, as I will now explore.

First, dys-appearance tends to arise when we are away, apart, from our ordinary mastery and health. There is the sense of privation, a reversal of a normal or desired state, which then provokes a bodily thematization.

In addition, at times of dys-appearance, the body is often (though not always) experienced as away, apart, from the self. Surfacing in phenomena of illness, dysfunction, or threatened death, the body may emerge as an alien thing, a painful prison or tomb in which one is trapped. As I will later discuss, these experiences of separation from, and opposition to, the body serve as one phenomenological basis for dualist metaphysics.[39] The experienced self is rent in two as one's own corporeality exhibits a foreign will.

This awayness of the body from its ideal or normal state and from the self-as-experienced is frequently based on spatio-functional and temporal sunderings within the body. The body can thus be away, apart, asunder, *from itself.* As Merleau-Ponty discusses, the intentional linkages between body and world and the synthetic unity of perceived objects all rest upon linkages within the lived body.[40] My two eyes integrate their powers to form a unified vision when, for example, I gaze at a vase. As I reach out to pick it up with my hands, vision is woven together with motility and touch. This synergy of bodily powers does not require the assistance of conscious will or intellection; it is a prethematic accomplishment. Nevertheless, as an accomplishment it can be threatened.

Breakdowns of sensorimotor synergy are one cause of dys-appearance. My right and left hands can fail to coordinate properly and the vase goes crashing to the floor. Or I may knock the vase over due to a visual mis-judgment. My attention is brought back to my bodily performance when I act in such an uncoordinated fashion.

The prethematic linkages that weave together visceral functions can also come apart. Such is often the case in disease. A specific organ, rather than serving the rest of the body, manifests an independent pat-tern. This may be due to a physiological failure, the invasion of external agents, or a cancerous overgrowth of autonomous cells. An organ sud-denly goes its own way, failing to perform its required role in proper coordination with others. One's body falls away, apart, from itself. Hegel thus characterizes a disease state:

> the system or organ establishes itself in isolation, and by persisting in its particular activity in opposition to the activity of the whole, obstructs the fluidity of this activity, as well as the process by which it pervades all the moments of the whole.[41]

This brings about a moment of negation within the organism:

> As a result of this susceptibility, there is a build up of a single aspect which does not accommodate the inner power of the organism, and the organism then exhibits the opposed forms of being and self, the self being precisely that for which the negative of itself has being.[42]

In experiential terms, one becomes aware of the recalcitrant body as sep-arate from and opposed to the "I." Yet as Hegel correctly points out, this arises from an opposition *within* the organism, not between it and an ontologically separate thing. The self that takes note of the body re-mains a moment of the organism, an *embodied* self. As I look down on a paralyzed limb I may be struck by the alien nature of embodiment. But I still use my eyes in looking down, my nervous system in thought, my other limbs in compensation for the paralyzed one. Gazing upon the body-object is a body-subject, though the physicality of the latter may remain tacit.

The body can grow away, apart, from itself not only through spatio-functional but temporal divisions. In addition to the synergic coopera-tion of organs, bodily intentionality rests upon continuities asserted across time. If my perceptual apparatus were transforming at every mo-ment, I could not know if perceived changes lay in the world or in myself. Only the structural stability of my body allows it to be an as-sumed basis from which I respond to an eventful world. This relative stability is true not only of my anatomical structure but of the mass of

skills and functional tendencies I incorporate. Only by virtue of my habitual action patterns can I tacitly inhabit the world.

When my embodiment radically diverges from the habitual, dys-appearance is likely to result. Sickness exemplifies not only a spatio-
functional but a temporal *écart*. When sick, the body changes, exhibiting novel sensations and altered capacities. In the face of such a
transformation I can no longer take the body for granted. This dys-
appearance by virtue of temporal discontinuity can also characterize
normal phases of life. In puberty and old age, one's body structure, appearance, and abilities undergo significant alterations. As such, greater
attention is often paid to the body at these times. The teenager looks for
physical changes in the mirror. The aging seek to adjust to unaccustomed limitations. In the middle years, women's bodies, more than
men's, also stand out as a place of transformation. Marked shifts occur
near and at the time of menstruation, yielding a heightened attention to
the physical. And in the progression of pregnancy, every month the
woman's body undergoes important changes. Using Merleau-Pontian
language, Young describes pregnancy as follows:

> My automatic body habits become dislodged, the continuity between my
> customary body and my body at this moment is broken. . . . In pregnan-
> cy my pre-pregnant body image does not entirely leave my movements
> and expectations, yet it is with the pregnant body that I must move.[43]

Young characterizes the pregnant woman as a "split subjectivity," both
one with the fetus and separate, locating herself in the eyes but also the
trunk, dwelling in both pregnant and prepregnant body images. Her
body is in the *dys* state, to use the Latinate sense: doubled, away, asunder
from itself.

There are possible dangers in assimilating such situations to the
model of dys-appearance. Phenomena such as aging, puberty, menstruation, and pregnancy are a normal and necessary part of the life
cycle. They are not in themselves dysfunctional or alienating. As such
they should not be associated with the notions of "bad" or "ill" that com-
prise part of the Greek meaning of *dys*. As Young forcefully argues, it is
only adult males in the middle years of life who experience health as an
unchanging state.[44] From this standpoint any noticeable changes do indeed signal disruption and dysfunction. However, for the young and the
aged, for adult women as opposed to men, normal body functioning
includes regular and even extreme bodily shifts. Cultural prejudices
lead us to forget or devalue such changes. Old age is frequently equated
with deterioration. Pregnancy and childbirth tend to be subsumed into
the medical paradigm as if they were dysfunctional states.[45] Yet, as

Gadow[46] points out in the former instance, and Young in the latter,[47] aging and pregnancy can be times in which one develops a new closeness to and valuation of one's body.

Nonetheless, aspects of this heightened body awareness can be understood according to the model of dys-appearance. While bodily states of rapid change need not be dysfunctional, they are indeed problematic. This might be seen as analogous to the time of mastering a new skill. The pregnant woman must attend to her body as its new functions and shape require alterations in patterns of movement, diet, sleep, etc. The very temporal and spatio-functional unity of her body are called into question. The aging person must adjust to a multitude of physical changes, while the young person reaching puberty struggles with a gawky body and a cracking voice, or the budding of breasts and the onset of menstruation. The assumption of a novel body renders problematic what was previously tacit.

Moreover, such states frequently do include moments of discomfort and dysfunction, though this hardly characterizes them as a whole. There is the morning sickness of early pregnancy, the uncomfortable and impeding bulk that comes later, all culminating in delivery pains. Puberty, in the case of women, brings with it the discomfort of menstrual cramps. Aging is often accompanied by a progressive loss of function and susceptibility to diverse aches and illnesses. All such phenomena play a part in bringing the body to dys-appearance at such times.

Beginning from etymology, I have thus catalogued the diverse ways in which the dys-appearing body is away, apart, asunder. The body emerges at times when it is away from an ordinary or desirable state, as in times of pain and disease. The body then may be experienced as away, apart, from the "I." This can arise from a loss of normal functional synergy, such that bodily organs operate apart from each other in an uncoordinated fashion. Through processes of change the momentary body may also grow away, apart, from the habitual body.

Thus, the presencing of the body in dys-appearance is still a mode of absence—etymologically, "to be away." In the modes of disappearance previously addressed, the body is away from direct experience. This could be called a *primary absence*. It is this self-effacement that first allows the body to open out onto a world. In dys-appearance the body folds back upon itself. Yet this mode of self-presence constitutes a *secondary absence*; the body is away from the ordinary or desired state, from itself, and perhaps from the experienced "I." This presence is not a simple positivity. It is born from the reversal, from the *absence of an absence*.

In characterizing bodily absence another complemental series emerges, which supplements those previously discussed. As a gestalt structure, the surface body disappears both as focal origin of and background to the sensorimotor field. When enlarging our perspective to include the body as a whole, we find it rendered tacit not only through these surface modes but through the depth disappearance of the visceral. These two complemental series, focal-background, surface-depth, account for the body's tendency to withdraw. However, in further extending our perspective to include thematic body experience, a third complemental series can be identified: that between disappearance as a whole and dys-appearance. No longer absent *from* experience, the body may yet surface as an absence, a being-away *within* experience. Health and illness can be taken as examples of the two complemental poles. Both exhibit an element of alienation from the body. In the case of health, the body is alien by virtue of its disappearance, as attention is primarily directed toward the world. With the onset of illness this gives way to dys-appearance. The body is no longer alien-as-forgotten, but precisely as-remembered, a sharp and searing presence threatening the self. One is a mode of silence, the other a manner of speech, yet they are complementary and correlative phenomena.

It would be a mistake to equate all modes of bodily thematization with dys-appearance. I may notice not only painful but neutral or pleasurable coenesthesias. I revel in the strength of my body during a race and the glow of well-being and relaxation that follows. I can look down at my arms and legs whenever I so choose and often do so inadvertently. I reach out to touch myself in a comforting way. I check a passing mirror to see how I look, making sure all is in order. In meditation I set aside times where I carefully follow my breath. There are a limitless variety of situations in which we experience or take action upon our body in the interest of enjoyment, self-monitoring, cultivating sensitivity, satisfying curiosity, or for no particular reason at all.

Yet, while episodes of dys-appearance exert no hegemony over the field of body awareness, I would argue that there is something that sets them apart and renders them unusually significant; they exhibit what I will term a character of "demand." Other sorts of bodily thematizations have a certain optional nature. I can choose to glance in a mirror or not, to develop the art of introspecting on my breath, or to simply remain oblivious to such things. Neutral, pleasurable, and theoretical self-explorations are of the sort to be volitionally pursued or neglected according to personal and social preferences. However, instances of dys-appearance demand attention. I am seized by a powerful pain or illness in a way that is unavoidable. The sensory intensity, the disruption of world relations, the telic demand for interpretation and problem resolution, all combine to compel awareness. As such, a heightening of body-focus at times of suffering and disruption, or of pregnancy and the acquisition of novel skills, will constitute something of a phenomenological invariant abiding across the range of individual and cultural differences.

Moreover, such phenomena place upon us not only an attentional but an existential demand. Our self-interpretation, importantly tied to the appearance and integrity of the body, is thrown into question at times of puberty, pregnancy, and aging. So too with serious illness, which can threaten our most cherished projects and reorganize our experience of world. These are moments of impending birth or death, devastation or renewal, calling forth deep-seated responses.[48] Neutral kinesthetic, visual, and tactile self-experiences may play as crucial a role in the construction of our body image, but they do not place upon one the same demand for an affective and metaphysical wrestling with embodiment. Hence, it is no coincidence that many philosophical and theological interpretations of the body have centered upon experiences of dys-appearance—disease, death, error, uncontrollable lust. Such experiences cry out for interpretation and control. Yet I will later suggest that this focus on dys-appearance has helped skew our cultural reading of the body toward the negative.

The Other

In concluding my phenomenology of dys-appearance it is necessary to discuss the pivotal role of the Other. There are two compelling reasons for this turn. First, my account would simply be incomplete without emphasizing the import of intersubjectivity. I have heretofore focused largely on the apprehension of the body from the first-person perspective. However, we are never proto-solipsists left to construct a body image in isolation. My awareness of my body is a profoundly social thing, arising out of experiences of the corporeality of other people and of their gaze directed back upon me. Am I fat or thin, beautiful or ugly, clumsy or agile? My self-understanding always involves the seeing of what others see in me. If it is to be adequate then, my category of dys-appearance must address intersubjective modes.

Moreover, I must discuss such modes in order to frame my account in relation to the phenomenological literature. Within this literature, bodily objectification and alienation have often been understood to result primarily from the look of the Other. This foreign gaze may first be internalized through the encounter with one's mirror image, as Lacan describes,[49] or in the actual confrontation with other people that Sartre discusses. In stressing the role of dys-appearance as provocateur of body awareness, I have advanced an alternative hypothesis. This hypothesis must prove itself capable of both incorporating the strengths and exposing the insufficiencies inherent in previous accounts. I will briefly attempt this, using Sartre as interlocutor.

For Sartre there is no true thematization of one's body prior to the encounter with the Other. The body as being-for-itself is always the "passed by in silence,"[50] a point of view upon the world that I *exist* without directly apprehending. At this stage even my pains are experienced through the world,[51] my illness suffered rather than known.[52]

With the introduction of the Other all is transformed. I now "experience the revelation of my being-as-object; that is, of my transcendence as transcended."[53] I come to thematize my body explicitly as an object, a tool among other tools or a collection of organs. This sense of myself as object correlatively brings about an undermining of my subjective possibilities. There is an "alienating destruction and a concrete collapse of *my* world which flows toward the Other and which the Other will reapprehend in *his* world."[54] We experience this in phenomena such as shyness and embarrassment.[55] Sartre's most famous example, though introduced prior to the explicit discussion of the body, is that of a man looking through a keyhole.[56] Initially the voyeur is simply lost in the world he regards, without reflective self-awareness. Suddenly he hears footsteps and apprehends his own position through the Other's look. His own project is truncated; he now stands pinned to his place, exposed and ashamed. Insofar as the Other is a subjectivity, the voyeur's own subjectivity is undermined.

How then does my discussion provide a tool both for criticizing this account and recognizing its points of validity? First, I have suggested that an explicit thematization of the body can arise independently of the Other's gaze. There are physical experiences such as pain, exhaustion, and illness that bring about the emergence of the body as explicit object. Corporeal alienation does not come to be solely through the social confrontation but from within the body-for-me. This thesis, argued as well by authors such as Zaner[57] and van den Berg,[58] need not be further elaborated here.

Second, I would suggest that Sartre's examples, far from revealing the general nature of being-with-Others, illustrate only a certain sort of encounter: precisely one marked by *dys-appearance*. To make this point, I will begin with a counterexample to those presented by Sartre.

I am walking in the forest with a friend. As we stroll we point out various things to one another: the color of the leaves, a passing bird, the changing of the seasons. I adjust to my friend's pace and she to mine. I find myself enjoying things more and in a different way than when I had come alone. We speak of other topics beside the scenery: of politics, mutual friends, movies each has seen. But then we lapse into silent enjoyment of our surroundings.

In such a situation, it is clear that being-with-another need not undermine bodily transcendence. We transcend together to a common world, sharing the forest in which we walk. My own subjectivity does not force the Other into the position of object, nor vice versa. We are cosubjectivities, supplementing rather than truncating each other's possibilities. I come to see the forest not only through my own eyes but as the Other sees it. Via gestures and word descriptions she opens me up to things I did not previously perceive. This process continues, on a more abstract level, as I hear her speak of mutual friends or movies I have not yet seen. My perspective upon the world is extended through hers.

I will call this phenomenon, which characterizes communicative sociality, *mutual incorporation.* I have discussed the body's ability to supplement its ecstatic powers through the incorporation of novel skills and tools. In an even more radical way we supplement our embodiment through the Other. Merleau-Ponty writes of how we discover in another's body:

> a miraculous prolongation of my own intentions, a familiar way of dealing with the world. Henceforth, as the parts of my body together comprise a system, so my body and the other person's are one whole, two sides of one and the same phenomenon, and the anonymous existence of which my body is the ever-renewed trace henceforth inhabits both bodies simultaneously.[59]

Through a natural empathy, one body takes up the affective responses of another. I feel sadness as I witness another's tears and am infected by his or her laughter. There is a further transmission of intentions allowed by the use of gestures and language. In mutual incorporation, each person's capacities and interpretations find extension through the lived body of the Other.

This is not to say that we ever merge into one. As Zaner notes, borrowing a term from Kierkegaard, I and another are always in a certain "dis-relationship," distanced from each other's perspective.[60] The limitation and particularization embodiment effects is the very ground of our separation. Yet it is also this separation that allows us to supplement one another's perspective. Mutuality is impossible in the absence of distance.

This mutuality cannot be construed as a derivative moment in the social dialectic. Merleau-Ponty points out that a baby will already imitate the gestures of adults prior to developing full awareness of its own body.[61] Intersubjectivity is intimately linked to such intercorporeity.[62] This primacy of mutuality is implicit even in Sartre's own account. He argues that the Other's gaze leads me to experience my own body as object. But this presupposes that, to some degree, I can see myself as others do. Only because my vision always incorporates that of other people could they have this power of negation over me. I put myself in their place, assume their perspective, just as they do mine. Hence, mutual incorporation is the necessary precondition of even the alienated gaze that Sartre describes. This mutuality never fully disappears, not even in the most objectifying encounter.

Nor is bodily objectification the necessary consequence of sociality. As discussed, when I walk with my friend through the forest I am not self-conscious about my movements and gestures nor focused on hers. Our bodies stand in cotransparency, ecstatically involved with a shared world. The structure of bodily disappearance is modified but fundamentally preserved in this being-with-another.

However, I can easily imagine a situation that would give rise to explicit body thematization. For example:

While walking with my friend in the forest I notice her surreptitiously sneaking glances at me. I become aware that she thinks that something is wrong with me: that my words, gestures and comportment are those of a seriously unbalanced man. As I describe a movie, she seems not to be imagining it along with me but focusing upon the strange way in which I talk. She apparently is looking for signs of my derangement. As I point out something in the forest, she seems struck by the outlandishness of my gestures, not by what I am gesturing toward.

In such a situation self-consciousness would be the norm. I would find myself monitoring my movements and tone of voice, trying overly hard to appear calm. We no longer transcend together to a common landscape or allow our moods and thoughts to mingle. The Other is interested in scrutinizing my intentions from outside, not taking them within. As Merleau-Ponty writes, in criticism of the Sartrian position:

The other person transforms me into an object and denies me, I transform him into an object and deny him, it is asserted. In fact the other's gaze transforms me into an object, and mine him, only if both of us withdraw into the core of our thinking nature, if we both make ourselves into an inhuman gaze, if each of us feels his actions to be not taken up and understood, but observed as if they were an insect's. This is what happens, for instance, when I fall under the gaze of a stranger. But even then, the objectification of each by the other's gaze is felt as unbearable only because it takes the place of possible communication. A dog's gaze directed towards me causes me no embarrassment. The refusal to communicate, however is still a form of communication.[63]

Mutual incorporation still takes place, but now precisely in the mode of refusal and disruption.

This disruption of communication gives rise to what I will term *social dys-appearance*. We have seen that dys-appearance results when the body is somehow away, apart, asunder, from itself, as in spatio-functional or temporal terms. In social dys-appearance, this split is effected by the incorporated gaze of the Other. But not just any gaze will bring about such a rupture; it is the objectifying gaze that refuses cotranscendence. As long as the Other treats me as a subject—that is, experiences *with* me to the world in which I dwell, mutual incorporation effects no sharp rift. But it is different when the primary stance of the Other is highly distanced, antagonistic, or objectifying. Internalizing this perspective, I can become conscious of my self as an alien thing.[64] A radical split is introduced between the body I live out and my object-body, now defined and delimited by a foreign gaze.

It is this structure of social dys-appearance, not of sociality as a whole, that Sartre so powerfully describes. As van den Berg writes:

> All the examples exposed in *L'être et le néant* to support this view are all equally misanthropic in character: a man peers through a keyhole at a scene not meant for his eyes and suddenly realizes that his reprehensible behavior is observed; another walks through a deserted street and hears behind him that an unknown person pulls aside the curtains to look silently after him. Sartre's look is the look from behind, the malicious look of an unknown person, the look that causes a shiver from neck to ankle.[65]

This split between the self and an alienated Other can inaugurate social dys-appearance.

As I have discussed, dys-appearance is hardly the sole mode of body awareness. This is true as well vis-à-vis the social realm. Van den Berg describes the encouraging, appreciative look that makes us aware of our embodiment in the mood of justification and acceptance.[66] I feel confirmed in my body by the lover's touch. However, the acceptance of mutuality most typically results in a tacit rather than thematized embodiment. We share moods, ideas, and experiences in cotranscendence. With ruptured communication the reverse is the case; disappearance can give way to dys-appearance.

As there are a variety of organic modes of dys-appearance—pain, fatigue, disability, etc.—so social dys-appearance can take many forms. In closing, I will sketch out a few such forms, without any attempt to be comprehensive. The social construction of body awareness is a huge and fascinating topic, touching as it does on questions of a historical, ethical, and political nature. Here I seek only to briefly suggest the relevance of the concept of dys-appearance to such concerns.

Sartre's example of a man looking through the keyhole illustrates that dys-appearance can be initiated by ethical distance or condemnation. Sartre's voyeur feels shame when discovered. The Other, it is assumed, would never do such a thing, would refuse to assume a similar posture and gaze. The voyeur becomes aware of his own position by virtue of this disrupted cosubjectivity. If the onlooker turns out to be a friend equally interested in taking a peek, the voyeur's self-consciousness would soon disappear. Their embodiments would no longer be away, apart, asunder, but interwoven in a common project.

Physical and cultural divergences can also bring about a dys-appearance. I most easily forget my body when it looks and acts just like everyone else's. However, walk into a party inappropriately attired, and self-consciousness returns. To take a more radical example, face-to-face with a New Guinea tribesman I should be much more aware of my appearance and dress than when wandering through my home town. Sometimes these physical/cultural divergences can be exaggerated by ideological agendas. In a racist society, a difference in skin color, trivial but highly noticeable, may lead to the assumption of the impossibility of communion. Hence the black often feels self-conscious wandering the white neighborhood, and vice versa. The disrupted sociality inherent in racism inaugurates a form of dys-appearance.

Dys-appearance also occurs in an aesthetic mode. I may be modeling for a painter or feel myself the object of a sexualized gaze. Such looks, depending upon the situation, might range from the enjoyable to the positively repulsive. Nonetheless they involve a certain rupture in mutuality. I become aware of myself as assumed into the Other's project, not as cosubjectivity. I may similarly become aware of my body as unsightly in the eyes of others. For example, I might be highly self-conscious concerning the size of my nose or the shape of my legs, such that a body-part magnifies itself to fill my field of awareness. This dys-appearance can then lead to a compensatory disappearance; I may attempt to forget my unattractive body by avoiding social occasions, mirrors, and the like, or fleeing into pure intellection.

Dys-appearance can also arise in a technical context, as when I am subjected to a doctor's physical exam. My body becomes a collection of organs, a mass to be studied and palpated. Corporeal self-consciousness, first provoked by the pain and dysfunction of my disease, now takes on a new dimension. Dys-appearance on the organic and social level can thus intertwine and be mutually reinforcing.

The example of the doctor-patient relationship touches on a further mode of social dys-appearance: that initiated by a discrepancy in power. When confronting another who has potential power over one's life and projects—the patient with the doctor, student with professor, prisoner with jailer—there is a tendency on the part of the powerless to a heightened self-awareness. The difference in power often precludes the assumption of cosubjectivity. It is not a matter of a reciprocal exchange of intentions, so much as one body submitting to the intentions of another. When a student gives an oral presentation under the teacher's evaluating eye, he cannot help a self-consciousness beyond that which he would feel with his peers. His own experience is not supplemented by the Other but, rather, supplanted. What the teacher sees is what really counts, and this alien look when incorporated leads to self-consciousness. Once again, social and organic dys-appearance intertwine; the student soon finds himself flushed and stammering.

Thus, the body is always a place of vulnerability, not just to biological but to sociopolitical forces. As Foucault writes:

> the body is also directly involved in a political field; power relations have an immediate hold upon it; they invest it, mark it, train it, torture it, force it to carry out tasks, to perform ceremonies, to emit signs.[67]

As Foucault explores in *Discipline and Punish,* the body is the setting of a "microphysics" of power.[68] Others can scrutinize and judge my actions, constrain my body in prison, inflict upon it pain or other forms of violation. They can regularize my movements as in an army drill or extract regimented labor. This susceptibility of the body to the Other's intentions, not just to illness and other organic forces, is a primary mechanism of dys-appearance. The prostitute, the tortured man, the assembly line worker, may each regard his or her body as if it were a thing. Their bodies have been taken away from them through the alienating projects of the Other.

Along these lines, it is notable that within our culture women tend to be more conscious of their bodies than men. To a limited extent this may result from biologically rooted dys-appearances as involved in the menstrual cycle or pregnancy. It is easier for adult men to ignore their largely unchanging bodies, while women receive more reminders of the visceral domain. However, much of this self-consciousness relates to a rupture in mutuality and a discrepancy of power. For, as Simone de Beauvoir explores, women assume the social role of Other, the "second sex."[69] It is the gaze, the projects of men that are culturally definitive. Hence women are not full cosubjectivities, free to experience from a tacit body. They must maintain a constant awareness of how they appear to men in terms of physical attractiveness and other forms of acceptability. Women are thus expected to pay meticulous attention to their surface appearance, including hairstyle, make-up, dress, weight, figure, and skin tone. This exhibits the principle of social dys-appearance; one incorporates an alien gaze, away, apart, asunder, from one's own, which provokes an explicit thematization of the body.[70]* Those with power in the situation need not experience reciprocal dys-appearance. For example, while a woman may become self-conscious walking in front of whistling longshoremen, they do not experience similar objectification in the face of her angry look back. As she is largely powerless in the situation, her perspective need not be incorporated; it can safely be laughed away or ignored.

I began this chapter with an examination of pain. Dys-appearance is operative in the most immediate and privatized of sensations. However, as is now clear, this structure plays a part in the broadest patterns of social behavior and power distribution. There is a reciprocal flow between such domains, the tracing out of whose complexities is a significant project; Foucault, Scarry, and a variety of feminist thinkers have done pioneering work here. Political power may operate through pain, as in the use of torture.[71] Conversely, pain may first render one available to power, as with the patient who checks into the hospital and finds herself at the mercy of its rules and hierarchies. Social dys-appearance may lead to biological dysfunction; a case in point is the current epidemic of anorexia nervosa, arising partially from cultural pressures upon women to achieve the "ideal body."[72] Or biological dysfunction may inaugurate social dys-appearance, such as is frequently experienced by the handicapped and disabled. The body is at once a biological organism, a ground of personal identity, and a social construct. Disruption and healing take place on all these levels, transmitted from one to another by intricate chiasms of exchange.

II
PHILOSOPHICAL
CONSEQUENCES

4

The Immaterial Body

The wonderful thing about language is that it promotes its own oblivion: my eyes follow the lines on the paper, and from the moment I am caught up in their meaning, I lose sight of them. The paper, the letters on it, my eyes and body are there only as the minimum setting of some invisible operation. Expression fades out before what is expressed, and this is why its mediating role may pass unnoticed, and why Descartes nowhere mentions it. Descartes, and *a fortiori* his reader, begin their meditation in what is already a universe of discourse. This certainty which we enjoy of reaching, beyond expression, a truth separable from it and of which expression is merely the garment and contingent manifestation, has been implanted in us precisely by language.

Maurice Merleau-Ponty, *Phenomenology of Perception*

A Diagrammatic Summation

In previous chapters I have presented several modes of corporeal absence. At any time, certain regions and functions of the body disappear from awareness. When the body does become the focus of thematic attention it is often as the result of another sort of absence: that of a desired or ordinary state and of the body's unproblematic unity with self.

These modes of absence arise directly out of the fundamental structure of embodiment. I have characterized the lived body as an ecstatic/recessive being, engaged both in a leaping out and a falling back. Through its sensorimotor surface it projects outward to the world. At the same time it recedes from its own apprehension into anonymous visceral depths. The body is never a simple presence, but that which is away from itself, a being of difference and absence.

I will employ a diagram to schematize the four modes of absence and the three complemental series I have discussed. The diagram takes the form of a "Necker cube," that is, one in which the perceptual gestalt can shift, bringing one face or another of the figure into the foreground.[1] This potential for perceptual reversal serves as a partial representation of the experiential reversals to which the body is prey. For example, in good health the face of disappearance (marked here by DIS) comes to the fore; body surface and depth disappear by virtue of their unproblematic operation. With an injury a sudden reversal takes place.

The face of dys-appearance (marked by DYS) stands out, as it is necessary to attend to a disrupted corporeality.

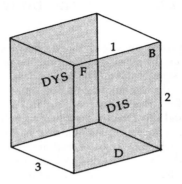

I will address the above diagram, beginning with the face of disappearance (DIS). The top horizontal axis, axis 1, represents the complemental series constituted by the body *surface*. As discussed, a complemental series is one in which a phenomenon emerges from the balanced operation of two etiological factors that stand in an inverse relationship such that the rising of one is necessarily linked to the decline of the other. In this case, the phenomenon referred to is the disappearance of the sensorimotor surface from conscious thematization. This results from the operation of two etiological factors, which I have termed focal and background disappearance (labeled F and B respectively on the diagram). At any given time, parts of the body surface constitute a focal origin from which I perceive or act, necessarily disappearing from the field they disclose. At the same time, other parts of the surface are forgotten by virtue of their background role relative to the gestalt of present functioning.[2]

I will characterize axis 1, the complemental series of the body surface, as *anatomically specified to a moderate degree*. To explain this notion I will return to the concept of a "phenomenological anatomy." I have engaged in a phenomenological description of lived experience and functioning. At the same time, my analysis has been anatomically guided. Different styles of existence are correlated with different physical regions of the body. That I live out my eyes in a dissimilar style from the way I do my spleen is associated with the anatomy of these organs, that is, their location, composition, and structural relations with other organs. Anatomy never totally specifies experience since the body is highly plastic, allowing for multiple modes of employment. However, the degree of freedom I have relative to different body regions is itself closely linked to anatomical factors; for example, I have far more freedom in how I choose to use my hands than I do in relation to my liver.

Whether a surface organ is employed in a focal or background role is only moderately specified by anatomy. The face, the hands, the mouth, the sensory organs, by virtue of their unique physical properties and functional importance, most frequently play a focal role in our communion with the world. Hence, such body areas tend to be assumed into focal disappearance. Conversely, the trunk and backside of the body, utilized in a largely supportive fashion, lend themselves to a background disappearance. However, this anatomical specification is incomplete, allowing a high degree of reversibility. The bodily distribution of these modes of disappearance depends upon patterns of individual and cultural usage and the vagaries of present action. I may employ my eyes to explore a landscape, but close them at the next moment to focus on audition. Eyes and ears exchange modes of disappearance. Focal and background disappearance thus dance across the body with rhythms of interchange and rapid reversal.

Such is not the case relative to axis 2 of the diagram. This represents the "vertical" dimension of the body, the complemental series constituted by the modes of surface disappearance on the one hand, and depth disappearance on the other hand. Depth disappearance (labeled D on the diagram) is the absence characteristic of organismic functions that proceed largely beneath the reach of direct perception and control. This form of absence, though operative to a certain extent throughout the body, predominates in relation to the visceral organs and certain temporal modes such as sleep or gestation. Unlike axis 1, the "horizontal" dimension of body surface, the "verticality" of axis 2 is *anatomically specified to a strong degree*. That is, the functional roles of body surface and depth cannot be easily exchanged. I can substitute an ear for an eye when attending to the world, but it would be impossible to substitute a pancreas. The depth location of the viscera, their relative paucity of sensory receptors and lack of voluntary musculature, specify the mode of disappearance they undergo. This specification is never absolute. For example, in a colostomy the gut is literally brought to the surface. Biofeedback or yogic training bring about their own forms of surfacing, fostering our awareness of, and control over, visceral processes. But the necessity of surgical intervention, technological incorporations, or highly disciplined training bears testimony to the difficulty of reversing surface and depth.

When corporeal function becomes problematic, all such modes of surface and depth disappearance can give way to the body's emergence as thematic object. This is represented in the above Necker cube by the coming to the fore of the face of dys-appearance (DYS). (These moments of disruption, when the body is away from its ordinary or desired state, are by no means the only times the body is thematized; this diagram is not meant to portray a complete phenomenology of the body but simply its modes of "absence" or awayness.) The diagrammatic face of dys-appearance covers the entirety of focal, background, and depth regions of embodiment, for all such regions can dys-appear. I may feel pain, for example, in my hands or my backside or my gut. Hence, axis 3, the complemental series constituted by the modes of bodily disappearance on the one hand, and on the other hand, the mode of dys-appearance, is *anatomically specified to a limited degree*. Almost any organ in the body can shift from a tacit to a problematic and experienced state. There may be rapid reversals as, for example, when a pain comes and goes. However, while anatomical specificity is limited relative to this complemental series, it still plays an important role. Certain visceral regions, such as the parenchyma of the liver and lung, are highly resistant to any thematic perception. They thus dwell irreversibly on the side of disappearance. Moreover, the character of dys-appearance differs markedly relative to different spatio-functional regions. The intrusiveness of the arthritic's hands, which grow subtly more painful, clumsy, and recalcitrant, bears little resemblance to the callings of an upset gut.

My summary diagram thus portrays the relationship of three complementary series, each one represented as the axis of a cube. It is important to note that rather than simply being correlative in structure, each complemental series builds upon the previous one. In dialectical fashion, the entirety of every complemental series except for the last is taken up as one polar extreme of a new series. Thus, the operation of focal and background regions defines the possibilities of surface disappearance. However, when viewing the body as a whole, the surface modes constitute but one general style of absence to be juxtaposed with that of the prepersonal depths. Finally, all such modes of disappearance still show but one way in which the body is absent, to be contrasted with the operation of dys-appearance.

Historical Dividends

At this point my work could well conclude. I have explored a limited phenomenological domain and sketched out its principle lines of forces. But if I were to abandon the project here much of its significance would remain implicit. For such a project is not enclosed within itself but is always situated within the broader discourse that constitutes the history of philosophical ideas. To ignore this in a fit of modernism would be to squander certain dividends that any phenomenological study can yield.

Such dividends are twofold. First, a search for the essential structures of lived experience frequently serves a critical function, yielding grounds for challenging previous philosophical positions. Merleau-Ponty's perceptually-based critique of intellectualism and empiricism is one case in point.[3] Indeed, the phenomenology of embodiment has so often been used as a way to attack previous positions, particularly Cartesian dualism and its rationalist and mechanist sequelae, that such a critique is more assumed than explicitly argued for in this work. I consider the territory as largely won by previous combatants.

Thus, I choose to focus instead on the second dividend that phenomenology can yield relative to the history of ideas, one all too often neglected. This could be called the *reconstructive* function. Any historical metaphysics that exhibits an enduring power and persuasiveness must, I would argue, have a meaningful phenomenological core. That is, it must describe and provide an interpretation for a range of significant human experiences. Though such experiences may remain hidden beneath a superstructure of abstractions and reifications, they can be reconstructed by a phenomenological rereading.

This reconstruction in turn serves two important functions. First, it buttresses the moment of criticism. To merely cite counterevidence to a previous philosophical position never really breaks its hold over our consciousness as long as its own domain of evidences is not admitted or explained. It is difficult, for example, to effectively challenge mind-body dualism unless its kernel of truth is recognized; there are, indeed, times in which the self is experienced as involving a mind-body opposition. Let it then be assumed that the philosophers of other centuries or persuasions are not dolts. One's own position will be most persuasive if it can provide an explanation, derived from its own internal presumptions, for why intelligent people would have found it plausible or even compelling to hold a contrasting view.

Furthermore, this phenomenological reconstruction not only strengthens the critique but institutes a project of reclamation. Reinterpreted in the guise of proto-phenomenology, the insights of a dualist such as Descartes no longer need be dismissed or used simply as a foil. A living fruit rests within its overly hard ontological husk. If one can strip that husk away, no longer adhering to strict systems of metaphysical opposition, one discloses a vibrant speech concerning human experience, and such phenomena as perception, thinking, knowledge and error, health and disease, embodiment and mortality. Metaphysics then is no longer that which is simply to be bracketed preliminary to a presuppositionless phenomenology. Rather, it provides a rich set of life-world descriptions and examples, of clues to guide our wanderings through the maze of experience.

In these last chapters I will focus specifically upon the work of Descartes as an exemplary site for this phenomenological rereading. I choose him for two reasons. First is his overwhelming importance in determining contemporary categories of the self. Whether it is the dualistic presumptions that guide everyday thought or the mechanistic worldview that still dominates much of science, we are all to a certain extent Cartesians in this culture, either willingly or struggling to get free. Second, he is chosen for his significance as the interlocutor most frequently addressed and excoriated by theorists of the lived body. As suggested above, the next logical step is not to simply criticize Descartes's worldview but to provide a phenomenologically-informed account of how he could have arrived at it and what it has to teach us.

In this chapter I will explore Descartes's characterization of the rational mind as immaterial. I will argue that one origin of this doctrine is to be found in the disappearances of the lived body I have charted out. Because the body is a tacit and self-concealing structure, the rational mind can come to seem disembodied. In the next chapter I will turn to the paradigm of the body often counterposed to this incorporeal mind. I will explore a variety of negative images with which the body comes to be associated, including those of error, disease, and death. Here, I will suggest, the phenomenon of dys-appearance plays a pivotal role. The tendency to thematize the body particularly at times of disruption helps establish an association between corporeality and its dysfunctional modes. The body is seen not only as Other to the self, but as a definite threat to knowledge, virtue, or continued life. Dualism thus reifies the absences and divergences that always haunt our embodied being.

The Place of Mind

I will begin by addressing Descartes's account of the physical location of mind. His portrait of mind-body dualism demands not only a functional analysis, as I will later pursue, but an analysis according to anatomy. The anatomical place of the mind is, for Descartes, in the strictest sense, nowhere. The mind as immaterial, a substance entirely opposed in nature to *res extensa,* has no extension or location in space. Such is demanded by Descartes's metaphysics. However, while this metaphysics serves certain theological and scientific purposes, it is inadequate for grounding a physiological psychology. There is as yet no accounting for that association of a particular mind with a particular body which establishes personal identity and unity.

Descartes is thus led to qualify his doctrine of the placelessness of mind. As he writes to Hyperaspites, "The mind is co-extensive with an extended body even though it has itself no real extension in the sense of occupying a place and excluding other things from it."[4] According to this notion, most clearly advanced in *The Passions of the Soul*, "the soul is united to all the portions of the body conjointly," such "that we cannot, properly speaking, say that it exists in any one of its parts to the exclusion of the others."[5] In a letter to Elizabeth[6] and in his *Reply to the Sixth Set of Objections*,[7] Descartes compares this model to that of gravity. Just as one conceives that gravity, while able to exert all its force through any single point, is coextensive with the entirety of a heavy body, so is the soul in relation to the human body.[8]

According to Descartes, this distributed soul correlates with the synthetic unity of the body in which it resides. Our physical organs are so intimately interrelated that "when any one of them is removed, that renders the whole body defective."[9] The continued presence of soul ultimately depends not on any particular body part but on the preservation of the overall union of its assembled organs.[10] The principle of a distributed soul is also implicit in some of Descartes's discussions of cognition.[10] For example, in letters to Meysonnier[11] and Mersenne, Descartes suggests that we should conceive of memory as found not only in the brain but elsewhere in the body:

> I think that all the nerves and muscles can serve it, too, so that a lute player, for instance, has a part of his memory in his hands: for the ease of bending and disposing his fingers in various ways, which he has acquired by practice, helps him to remember the passages which need these dispositions when they are played.[12]

In advancing this doctrine of a distributed soul or mind (for he fully identifies the soul with the mind),[13] Descartes engages in a proto-phenomenology. That is, he seeks to express and account for our experience of the synthetic nature of lived embodiment. Just as gravity can exert its force through a point of mass, so can an individual organ be made focal in the body gestalt. When I swing an axe, for example, all my energy floods out through my arms. However, at the same time, this swing is supported by my body working as an integrated gestalt; my purposiveness most properly resides in the body as a whole. Moreover, as Descartes recognizes, there are loci of intelligent ability and memory distributed throughout the body. Practiced hands can tie a knot that words could not explain. A doctor's trained ear can recognize the arrhythmia inaudible to the book-fed student. In the broadest sense, mentality is indeed distributed throughout the lived body. Descartes's notion of a distributed soul expresses this insight well.

However, this is not his primary model. It appears nowhere in the *Meditations*. In *The Principles of Philosophy*[14] and even in *The Passions of the Soul*, the doctrine of distributed soul is introduced mainly as a qualification to his central point, "that there is a small gland in the brain in which the soul exercises its functions more particularly than in the other parts."[15] According to this well-known doctrine of *limited* mind-body interactionism, the mind principally perceives and acts upon the body through one place, the pineal gland, a small portion of the brain. Only here does soul directly exercise its power:

> And the whole action of the soul consists in this, that solely because it desires something, it causes the little gland to which it is closely united to move in the way requisite to produce the effect which relates to this desire.[16]

Only here does the soul directly receive corporeal impressions:

> It is however easily proved that the soul feels those things that affect the body not in so far as it is in each member of the body, but only in so far as it is in the brain.[17]

In *The Principles of Philosophy* Descartes refers to three classes of phenomena as evidence for this localized view of mind-body interaction.[18] First, certain maladies, along with sleep, which affect the brain alone, disorder or take away from us the use of the senses. Second, if there is nerve obstruction between certain body parts and the brain, all sensation in those parts is lost. Third, we sometimes feel pain as though it were in certain of our members, when the true cause lies in other regions through which the nerves pass on their way to the brain. Descartes himself wrote of having known a girl who complained of pains in her hand and arm long after these had been amputated for gangrene.[19]

Thus, just as the doctrine of distributed mind accounts for a certain range of lived phenomena, so certain experiences, both of ordinary life and unusual medical contingency, provide support for this more localized view. Moreover, to Descartes's list of phenomena, testifying to the central role of the brain in mediating consciousness, many others could now be added. Through contemporary technologies it is possible to witness the motor and perceptual results of direct brain stimulation and map out the brain-wave activity and neurotransmitter release which accompany diverse states of consciousness. While Descartes's conjectures concerning the pineal gland in particular have long since been discredited, his focus upon the brain as a principal seat of mentality is buttressed by a convincing variety of evidence. This raises an important point for my exploration of bodily disappearance. If an understanding is to be reached as to why mind has been portrayed as an immaterial, transparent essence, it is necessary to address that bodily organ most central to mind's operation: the brain.

Phenomenology and the Brain

The brain has been almost totally ignored in previous treatments of the lived body. When discussed, it is often in a polemical context: "It is man who thinks, not the brain," writes Erwin Straus.[20] Physiologically defined as a set of nerves, synapses, chemical discharges, the brain, he argues, should not be confused with the experiencing subject. Nor is it the object of experience; I see the trees and sky, not the neuronal firings that accompany this perception. In the wake of its reductionist employments, any mention of the brain comes to imply an eradication of lived experience in favor of its causal/physicalistic correlates.

This need not be the case. The brain belongs exclusively to causal analysis only if phenomenologists refuse its discussion. As with any other corporeal structure—the eye, the mouth, the hand—the brain can be understood not only physicalistically but as an organ of the lived body, a structure of possibility opening onto the world.

The reason for the phenomenological neglect of the brain is readily apparent; this organ is almost never present as an object of direct perception or control. Unlike the body surface, visible to self and Other, the brain rarely makes an appearance in the life-world. Admittedly, it is available in certain limited ways; we see brains at autopsy, through diagnostic imaging techniques, or pictured in textbooks. There is a fund of intersubjective experience here that inevitably surpasses any first-person awareness. Yet in the everyday life-world it is highly unusual to encounter a brain.

However, as my study has suggested, disappearance is a crucial feature of all lived embodiment. The absence of body regions from thematic perception has been shown to be necessary to their operation. The almost complete disappearance of the brain may thus attest not to its irrelevance but to its centrality relative to lived experience. Far from resisting a phenomenological treatment, this absent-brain cries out for one. I will account for the phenomenon by referring to modes of bodily disappearance previously discussed. This disappearance of the brain, principal organ of mentality, will provide a first clue to the seeming disembodiment of mind.

In his book *Body Image and the Image of the Brain,* Gorman notes that one's image of one's own brain, unlike most parts of the body, is not governed by direct perception. He writes:

> while the hand's appendages, the fingers, enable us to feel the hand, and the eye may see itself, one's own brain has not been touched, nor has it been felt, even by the most curious. Instead, the brain lies encased within the cranial vault. . . . Not only are we denied the possibility of touching our own brains, but also the brain itself is impervious to touch. The matter of the brain itself, in alert and conscious patients, may not only be touched and stimulated electrically, but also may be suctioned, cut or cauterized without the patient perceiving that his brain has been touched or instrumentated.[21]

Here is a form of depth disappearance. Like my visceral organs, my brain is enfolded within the depths of my body, hidden away from my exteroceptive powers and those of others. And like the most reticent of viscera, such as liver or spleen, the brain is absent from interoception as well. It is "impervious to touch," as Gorman writes. (Headaches and other cranial sensations involve the surrounding meninges or musculature, not the brain substance itself.) It was, in fact, such evidence that led Aristotle to mistakenly infer the exclusively visceral nature of the brain:

> That is has no continuity with the organs of sense is plain from simple inspection, and is still more clearly shown by the fact, that, when it is touched, no sensation is produced; in which respect it resembles the blood of animals and their excrement.[22]

As with other visceral organs, this sensory lack is tied to a motor disappearance from self and world. While I may suspect that every thought or action correlates with changes in my brain state, I experience no direct control over the organ any more than I do over my liver. I cannot, for example, simply will an adjustment in my hypothalamic functioning. Nor is the brain available to the direct action of the outside world. As Freud writes:

> This little fragment of living substance is suspended in the middle of an external world charged with the most powerful energies; and it would be killed by the stimulation emanating from these if it were not provided with a protective shield against stimuli.[23]

Like the viscera, the brain requires this encasement in bodily depths. This serves a protective function as well as allowing for the operation of mediating structures. The brain is fitted neither to experience nor act upon the world directly, but relies upon the intercession of a sensori-motor apparatus.

Thus, the brain shares with the viscera a depth disappearance, a withdrawal from the circuit of direct perception and control. This visceral connection is not only a phenomenological but a physiological fact; the brainstem in particular is intimately connected with visceral processes, playing a key role in governing respiration, circulation, and body temperature, along with a host of other autonomic functions. Such intricate regulations proceed largely without the supervision of the conscious "I." They unfold according to the anonymous logic of the "it can."

THE BRAIN AND SURFACE DISAPPEARANCE

The brain, of course, does far more than modulate visceral functions. It lies at the seat of embodied thought, sensory experience, and voluntary movement. This presents a seeming paradox. That organ which subtends embodied consciousness is itself unavailable to conscious apprehension. Yet this disappearance is nothing but the radicalization of a phenomenon already discussed: the focal disappearance of the surface body. That from which I perceive and act necessarily resists my thematization. As I gaze upon the world, I cannot see my own eyes. The disappearance of brain is an expression of this same principle. (Indeed, the retina and optic nerve are embryologically an outpocketing of the wall of the brain.) Not only are my own eyes invisible to me, but so too my optic nerves and the visual cortex of my brain. For, taken as a group, these belong to the corporeal means from which I see and hence are not the object of this sight. Similarly, the several areas of the brain that govern movement, along with the nerves that innervate my hand, are not themselves thematized objects of my reach; they are part of the neurological grouping from which I reach. Another could observe my neuronal firings at such moments and draw the correlations. But my brain-as-lived is not yet an objectification. It is part of my ecstatic mode of access to the world. It thus recedes from my direct apprehension even as it grounds my experience.

This focal disappearance of the brain is more thorough than that of its allied surface organs. Such organs need be functionally tacit only within the particular range of experience in which they play a focal role and thus may be thematized in other ways and times. While the eye recedes in visual experience, it can always be touched. However, as that which subserves conscious experience and voluntary action in general, my brain is constantly playing a tacit role. There is no second organ of consciousness with which to observe the first.

Moreover, the brain is set apart from other ecstatic organs not only by the range but by the centrality of its tacit role. It is easier to thematize the more distal elements of a "from" structure. If I am poking something with a stick, I can switch my focus to the stick itself, feeling its impact upon my hand. More difficult, yet possible via an attentional shift, is to experience the tactile sensations strictly as modifications of my own hand. However, I cannot continue on indefinitely and experience directly the nerves in my hand or my somesthetic cortex. Ultimately there are elements so proximal within the "from" structure that they are irreversible for the subject, unavailable for being experienced "to." (Polanyi refers to these as subliminal stimuli and includes neural traces as an example.)[24] The nervous system lies at the very core of the experiencer. As such, it radically resists alienation and objectification.

THE BRAIN AND THE IMMATERIAL MIND

Our lived mentality cannot simply be equated with brain function but is ultimately distributed throughout the body. It is not the brain alone that formulates speech, turns a discerning eye upon the environment, moves intelligently to accomplish its projects. For this, mouth, eye, and limbs are needed as well, our entire corporeal presence taking in and acting upon the world. The lived body is mentalized through and through, all of its organs participating in a uniquely human intelligence.

However, one can, as does Descartes, speak of the brain as the principal bodily seat of mind. Not because it is somehow disconnected from other organs but precisely because it is connected with all, a node of synthesis wherein the different sensory channels are blended, perception gives rise to movement, volitional acts are coordinated with unconscious visceral changes. The brain (or more generally, the central nervous system) weaves the threads of a unified body. The brain is thus a microcosm of the whole body, participating in its chiasm of surface and depth. It might then be termed a *microchiasm*. The cerebral cortex, largely involved with conscious and volitional processes, chiasms with the brainstem, central to vegetative homeostasis. The brain's neurons are derived from ectoderm, the tissue of the embryological surface, yet the brain is enfolded into bodily depths. The brain is a functional and anatomical microchiasm.

As such, the brain partakes of *all modes* of body disappearance, and each to a heightened form. Its interoceptive withdrawal is so complete, along with the threat to life that would be caused by its exposure, that the brain is hidden away as thoroughly as any viscus. Its central role in the "from" structure of perception and motility dictates a focal disappearance surpassing that of other surface organs. When combined, the outcome is an almost complete absence from experience.

This invisibility of the brain is one experiential source for the notion of the human mind as immaterial. Our principal organ of mentality seems nowhere to register in the physical world. When I look into the eyes of another, they are like windows that lead inward to a place of consciousness and desire. Yet this place continually escapes direct apprehension. As Merleau-Ponty writes, the seer "is always *a little behind* what the other sees,"[25] an invisibility receding beneath the visible eyes. This sense of mind-as-invisible is reinforced from the first-person perspective. I can no more discover from whence my acts and words emanate than can the Other. A song runs through my head. One thing "comes to mind" rather than something else. I discover I have finally mastered a skill. Different organs of my body seamlessly synthesize their motions. But I myself apprehend no material basis for this intelligence and coordination. My brain, as that which I exist from within, manifests no physical presence for me directly to know. I cannot get a distance on it, render it visible, for it is at the very hidden heart of me wherever I go. Human mentality can thus seem immaterial, disembodied, as if of another order of things. An experiential disappearance is read in ontological terms. Yet, as I have attempted to indicate, this disappearance arises precisely from the *embodied* nature of mind. The body's own structure leads to its self-concealment.

The Activity of Mind

My discussion of the notion of the "immaterial" mind has so far been anatomically guided. I have focused on the brain, an organ from which we live out our mentality. However, to further understand the roots of Cartesianism, I must turn to a more functional approach. That is, I must address the activities that have characteristically been attributed to mind. Not only certain organs but certain modes of action particularly efface their bodily roots.

For Descartes, "there is always one principal property of substance which constitutes its nature and essence, and on which all the others depend."[26] In the case of the substance of mind or soul, "thought" is the defining attribute. Yet this seemingly simple assertion masks a crucial ambiguity. Just as Descartes advances more than one doctrine concerning the place of soul, so its essential activity is characterized in differing ways. At times thought is equated with the field of consciousness as a whole, at other times, exclusively with the faculty of understanding.[27] As before, I will seek to mine this ambiguity for its power of phenomenological disclosure.

Mind as Consciousness

In perhaps the most famous passage of the *Meditations,* Descartes writes:

> But what then am I? A thing which thinks. What is a thing which thinks? It is a thing which doubts, understands, [conceives], affirms, denies, wills, refuses, which also imagines and feels.[28]

Descartes at first makes no distinction in essence between these differing forms of consciousness. They are all considered equally as modes of thought. As he writes in *The Principles of Philosophy,* "By the word thought I understand all that of which we are conscious as operating in us."[29] By employing this term to refer to willing and perceiving as well as abstract cognition, Descartes widens the notion of to think (*cogitare, penser*) well beyond that employed in colloquial or traditional philosophical usage.[30] As Richard Rorty discusses, a new idea thus enters the philosophical scene, that

> of a single inner space in which bodily and perceptual sensations . . . mathematical truths, moral rules, the idea of God, moods of depression, and all the rest of what we now call "mental" were objects of quasi-observation.[31]

From this perspective, thought is equated with conscious experience as such, and consciousness with the gaze of an immaterial mind.

This sense of human awareness as immaterial is facilitated and encouraged by bodily disappearance. Our conscious interaction with the world is sustained via a sphere of anonymous visceral functions: the beating of the heart, the kidney's filtration, a hundred other vital processes. Yet these processes are carried out unconsciously, wrapped in a depth disappearance. Because such processes recede from the phenomenal life-world, human consciousness may seem *causa sui,* intertwined with no material principle. And in addition to this withdrawal of the unconscious body, there is a self-effacement within the structure of consciousness. As I have discussed at length, my experiencing body is ecstatic, directed away from itself. That from which I perceive, my body is literally over-looked. It can thus seem as if the experienced world is arrayed before the gaze of a disembodied mind.

There is much in ordinary experience to undercut this presumption including, of course, the role of movement. The perceiver is always also an actor, reaching out to touch, turning to look, going toward or away from objects on the basis of pragmatic goals. This motor involvement with the world, while exhibiting its own ecstatic structure, is clearly physical in nature. Human awareness can seem most disembodied only when the deep connection between perception and movement is broken. And so it is for Descartes. According to his metaphysics, motion must always fall on the side of *res extensa*. It is an attribute of extended bodies, not of consciousness.[32] This ontological sundering allows consciousness to be modeled as a spectacle unfolding before a detached observer, one who is in the world but not of it.

VISION

This sundering of awareness and movement would seem implausible unless it also found roots within the living body. One bodily origin is suggested by the very metaphor of consciousness as "spectacle"—that is, the faculty of vision. As Jonas and Rorty discuss, the visual model of mind has played a determinative role in the Western tradition.[33] Plato describes *nous* as the "eye of the soul"[34] gazing upon the *eidos*—a term that, while understood as immaterial "form" or "idea," retains its etymological sense of "visible image." Similarly, Descartes refers to the intellect as an "eye of the mind."[35] Via the "light of nature" it is capable of perceiving ideas "clearly and distinctly."[36] As Rorty notes, "in the Cartesian model, the intellect *inspects* entities modelled on retinal images."[37]

Vision lends itself to such analogies with the intellect because of its great epistemological significance. Important essays by Jonas[38] and Straus[39] explore sight as the gnostic sense par excellence. It gives us in one glance a more comprehensive survey of the surrounding world, more detailed information about any particular object, more knowledge concerning the stable attributes of a thing, than does any other sense. Hearing, by contrast, reveals particular events, not definite objects, becoming, not being. But the "mind's" knowledge of a stable, copresent, external world is, indeed, largely derived from the eye. Thus, in a model such as Descartes's, which emphasizes the epistemological subject and regards truth as involved with definiteness and permanence, visual experience will be attended to above all others. It emerges as "the noblest and most comprehensive of the senses"[40] as Descartes writes at the beginning of the *Dioptrics,* his work devoted to vision.

However, it is precisely visual experience that lends itself most to an experience of disembodiment and the seeming detachment of perception from motility. In touch, sensation is clearly tied to physical movements. Touching begins as I reach out to contact the object, and the quality of sensation is elicited by my style of motion: for example, whether I stroke or press. This motor involvement is far less obvious with sight. In the fixed gaze, a vast spectacle presents itself without any perceptible movement on my part. The body's motility is placed in background disappearance. Moreover, as Jonas describes, sight involves a "dynamic neutralization" of experienced causation.[41] Due to the properties of light and the visual apparatus, one experiences no sense of physical force or impact exerted upon oneself by the viewed scene. Neither is this scene physically affected by one's gaze. Unlike the probing finger, the eye leaves its object of exploration unchanged. Jonas sees in such features of vision the birth of the notion of *theoria,* a detached rather than praxical relation to the world.[42] The body as the place of action and forceful interchange with the world for the moment fades away. This is intensified by the spatial distances sight opens, allowing the subject to dwell experientially far off. In touching, one's own body remains a proximate copresence with the touched, always immediately implicated. But visual awareness, as when I gaze upward to the stars, can focus trillions of miles away.

Through such attributes of relative immobility, dynamic neutralization, and spatial reach, sight, more thoroughly than any other perceptual mode, effaces its rootedness in the body. The viewer can seem to be an incorporeal awareness.

However, this effacement is never complete. The visual scene, like any field of perception, always contains within it implicit reminders of the body. The perspectival and limited nature of the spectacle, seen incompletely and from a particular angle, suggests a viewer localized in space, restricted by position and perceptual apparatus. The embodied nature of the subject is similarly suggested by the embodied nature of the perceptual object. As Descartes notes, sense experiences present themselves independently of my will and with a liveliness exceeding the productions of my own meditations.[43] Thus, I experience my sensory images as deriving from an external and very material world of rocks and houses and trees. The corporeality of the onlooker is correlatively implied; "like know like" was a plausible assumption for Descartes as for Plato and Aristotle. In the physical and perspectival nature of the perceived world I find ceaselessly suggested my own embodied participation.

There is then an experiential ambiguity to perception as exemplified by vision; it seems both to escape and inhere in a body. I would suggest that this is one root of Descartes's ambiguous position vis-à-vis perception's ontological status. On the one hand he regards perception as a mode of thought, and hence as belonging to *res cogitans.* However, Descartes also contends that in its full reality, perception necessarily involves the body. He is driven to define a broad class of phenomena "which should be attributed neither to mind or body alone, but to the close and intimate union that exists between the body and mind."[44] This category is said to include all sensory experience, "such as pain, pleasure, light and colour, sounds, odours, tastes, heat, hardness, and all other tactile qualities," along with appetites such as hunger and thirst and emotions such as anger, joy, sadness, and love. In a sense, Descartes is not a dualist as much as a trialist. Along with those functions which belong to mind or body taken separately, he attributes a class of psychological phenomena to the entity formed of their union.

There is thus a tension in Descartes's account of perception; it is taken up both qua mode of thought and as embodied phenomenon.[45] One source of this tension is clearly to be found in Descartes's multiplicity of scientific roles. As physicist he seeks to banish all residues of subjectivity from the material realm. Conversely, as psychophysiologist, he must acknowledge the interpenetration of mind and body. However, I have also tried to suggest a further source for this tension, one rooted in the life-world itself. Episodes of perceiving, particularly when vision is made paradigmatic, involve a strong element of bodily disappearance. They thus allow themselves to be modeled as dephysicalized events. Yet at the same time, such experiences include powerful reminders of the subject's corporeality, thus necessarily undermining this model. The body is phenomenologically both erased and asserted. Taken by themselves, such perceptual modes do not yield the sense of mind as fully disembodied.

Mind as the Understanding

One must then look elsewhere for the experiential core of this doctrine. If our sensory faculties do not constitute mind's immaterial essence, what if anything does? Descartes's answer is clear; it is the intellectual faculty of "understanding." The understanding is nothing less than the rational mind operating independently of all bodily influences. In the *Rules for the Direction of Mind,* Descartes first suggests that while the spiritual power of mind applies itself to corporeal impressions when perceiving, remembering, imagining, "if it act alone it is said to understand."[46] Similarly, in the *Meditations,* imagining is said to involve a turn toward the body, while in "pure intellection . . . mind in its intellectual activity in some manner turns on itself, and considers some of the ideas which it possesses in itself."[47]

Descartes understands this autonomy in a quite literal fashion. I earlier discussed his placing of mind in close association with the brain. However, if acts of intellection are fully independent of the body, they must proceed without reliance even upon cerebral traces:

> I have often also shown distinctly that mind can act independently of the brain; for certainly the brain can be of no use in pure thought: its only use is for imagining and perceiving.[48]

This notion that the intellectual soul is self-contained rather than dependent upon the "various dispositions of the brain" is reiterated in a 1639 letter to Mersenne.[49] Descartes goes so far as to distinguish between the two forms of memory, one bodily and one purely intellectual. When we think of corporeal things, particles are set in motion in the brain, leaving physical residues.[50] But the intellect contains a completely different sort of memory "which is certainly independent of the body."[51]

Descartes distinguishes the understanding from the imagination by virtue of the former's nonreliance on corporeal imagery. In his famous example of the "chiliagon" he argues that we can conceive of entities without forming a mental picture of them.[52] Certain immaterial things, such as God or the soul, he regards as simply impossible to represent via an image; they can only be conceived of by the abstract intellect.[53] For Descartes, this abstract, imageless thought constitutes the one mental activity that is completely disembodied.

Rorty[54] and Matson[55] have emphasized the important break between the Cartesian concept of mind and that of the ancient Greeks. They note that for the Greeks, unlike Descartes, sense-perception was not a form of "thought" but clearly belonged to the body. Only in intellectual reason is found the activity definitive of the human mind. However, as now can be seen, Descartes is not that distant in spirit from the ancients; he too establishes a strong linkage between the mind and a purified intellect. Just as Plato argues that one can never apprehend absolutes via any bodily sense, but must apply "pure and unadulterated thought to the pure and unadulterated object,"[56] so, for Descartes, the soul can only apprehend metaphysical notions and achieve clear and distinct knowledge via a reason freed from reliance upon the senses. Such a reason expresses the soul's incorporeal essence. To understand Descartes's doctrine of immaterial mind, then, one must turn to the phenomenon of intellectual thought.

Thinking is usually modeled by contemporary psychologists as employing a combination of language and pictorial imagery.[57] Of these, I will focus on the importance of language in shaping the Cartesian view of the understanding. I do this for two reasons, one internal, one external, to the Cartesian corpus.

First, Descartes himself specifically excludes thought involving pictorial imagery from pure intellect. As discussed, such thinking is consigned to the faculty of the imagination and is said to reflect corporeal influence. It is true that Descartes, in accord with the assumptions of his time and the demands of his metaphysics, also distinguishes ideas from their linguistic expression. However, he recognizes that pure ideas "are commonly associated with names,"[58] and that "we can scarcely conceive of anything so distinctly as to be able to separate completely that which we conceive from the words chosen to express the same."[59] Thus, Descartes suggests that the ideas of the understanding are more closely associated with language than with visual imagery.

Second, the key role played by language in structuring abstract thought is confirmed by psychological introspection and research. For example, Paivia distinguishes between the styles of thinking employed in concrete and abstract reflection. While visual imagery is used more when we think about concrete objects and events, abstract thought, which entails generalization, symbolic reasoning, and the integration of information not immediately available to the senses, is predominantly language-mediated.[60]

Thus, I will now turn attention to language and its modes of embodiment. I will first discuss the ways in which public uses of language, that is, speech and writing, involve structures of bodily disappearance. I will then show how this disappearance intensifies when language is interiorized into silent thought. Herein lies a clue to the seeming disembodiment of the intellect.

LANGUAGE AND THOUGHT

That language is a profoundly embodied affair is made evident by the example of language acquisition. As earlier discussed, prior to mastering a language I thematize *to* it as a foreign thing. I observe the spelling of words, listen to their sound, practice my pronunciation, and study rules of grammar. It is only via a process of incorporation that the language truly becomes mine. When proficient, I no longer thematize to the words but from them as an instrument of generating and receiving meaning. My eyes finally scan a book with comprehension. My mouth can now articulate what I want to say. The language, similar to any skill or tool, becomes a part of my bodily "I can." As Sartre writes, "Consciousness of the body is comparable to the consciousness of a *sign*. The sign moreover is on the side of the body; it is one of the essential structures of the body."[61]

The structural and material properties of the sign can be related back to this incorporative process. The sign is frequently understood according to a distinction between the signifier and its meaning or referent. Yet this division derives from the "from-to" structure of embodiment. In employing a sign I do not thematize its sheer physical presence (the signifier) but attend from it to that which is signified. The signifier thus undergoes a focal disappearance as it is incorporated. The double-sidedness of the sign, both material thing and self-transcending intention, derives from its use by the double-sided lived body.

Moreover, the signifiers employed in language are chosen so as to facilitate this bodily use. As Suzanne Langer writes:

> Another recommendation for words is that they have no value except as symbols (or signs); in themselves they are completely trivial. . . . A symbol which interests us *also* as an object is distracting. It does not convey its meaning without obstruction. For instance, if the word "plenty" were replaced by a succulent ripe, real peach, few people could attend to the mere concept of *quite enough* when confronted with such a symbol. . . . But little noises are ideal conveyors of concepts, for they give us nothing but their meaning. This is the source of the transparency of language on which several scholars have remarked. Vocables in themselves are so worthless that we cease to be aware of their physical presence at all, and become conscious only of their connotations, denotations, or other meanings.[62]

In other words, the nondistracting nature of the signifier facilitates its incorporation. That which does not demand attention-to can more easily be attended-from. The written word thus has no three-dimensional depth, takes up little space, and usually evidences no outstanding beauty in its shape. The spoken word is even more transparent, for it asserts no visible presence and fades away as soon as it is uttered. The body of the sign is thus self-effacing. It can seem an immaterial thing.

Similarly, the human body effaces itself in the use of language. The organs directly involved in receiving and generating signs are in focal disappearance. In reading, I do not attend to my eyes but from them. I do not attend to my mouth when speaking, or my ears when hearing, but from them to the articulated meanings. At the same time as these organs focally disappear, the rest of the body is often placed in background disappearance. The minimal materiality of linguistic signs demands only a minimal though intricate use of the body: small gestures of the writing hand, a swift scanning by the eyes, subtle movements of the lips and tongue. This serves an important function in the body economy, allowing for maximal speed and combinatory number in exchange for little expenditure of energy. Bertrand Russell makes this point in relation to speech: "there is no other way of producing a number of perceptively different bodily movements so quickly and with so little muscular effort."[63] The result is that language use is compatible with relegating most of the body to a merely supportive role. I forget my torso, the position of my legs, the panorama of the senses, as I concentrate here on my reading and writing. In listening to a friend I am "all ears." Other bodily regions recede into a tacit background.

So far, I have focused on the structures of disappearance common to spoken and written language. Both involve an effacement of the body of the sign and the body of the subject engaged with language. However, before proceeding onward, it is necessary to pause to recognize an important distinction. In speech, language remains closely wedded to its point of origin in the human body. Speech (excepting the question of recordings) happens in the immediate context of an embodied speaker and listener. Written language, on the other hand, brings with it a surplus detachment. For when written down, words and the ideas they express seem to develop a career independent of human bodies. Language, as concretized in the text, leaves behind its voice of origin, is able to live on through the centuries, to be instantiated unchanged in an indefinite number of locales.

Havelock[64] and Abram[65] have argued that this is one source for the Platonic notion of a realm of unchanging, disembodied Ideas. Ideation, as instantiated in writing, seems to have freed itself from the spatiotemporal limits of the body and to represent something independent and eternal. Correlative to this "disembodied" object of knowledge, it seems plausible to conjecture a disembodied knower. Havelock argues that the notion of intellectual soul, unknown in oral cultures, is crucially tied to the development of literacy.[66*] Given the profound distrust of writing expressed in the *Phaedrus,* it is ironic that literacy may have played a key role in provoking and supporting Platonic doctrines.[67]

However, the acts of writing and reading, involving an exteriorized, incarnated language, would not in themselves provide direct evidence of an interior, immaterial mind. It is when the abstract concepts of a literate culture are taken up into verbal thought that the subject most seems to be disembodied. For the bodily disappearance of the self reaches an extreme in such thought. The structures of effacement characteristic of public language use are further exaggerated when language turns inward. When engaged in inner monologue, even my hands and mouth, my eyes and ears, drop out of immediate employment. The sensorimotor organs that were used in speaking or reading are now placed in background disappearance with the rest of the body. I can think while sitting perfectly motionless, no corporeal activity whatsoever apparent to myself or to another. *It seems as if the thinker makes no use of a body.*

In fact, the body is still involved; the use of signs ever remains its province. As philosophers, historians, and psychologists have suggested, interior speech is logically and temporally dependent upon speech as employed in the public setting.[68] Thought first arises in a context of material signifiers and social practices. Nor does the interiorization of language free it from its inherence in the physical. Famous experiments by Jacobson showed that minute movements of the vocal apparatus accompany our thinking.[69] We remain unaware of these subvocalizations due to their subtlety and hidden location. Moreover, thought involves the brain's unseen activity. Due to the focal and depth disappearance of the brain, I do not experience its role in subserving my thought, nor do those around me. Thinking simply seems to come, involving no material substructure.

In conjunction with this disappearance of the body of the thinker is an intensified disappearance of the sign-body. (As the sign is an incorporated structure, these are in fact two aspects of a single phenomenon.) There is no externally audible sound, no visible mark, in the inner monologue. Its seeming disembodiment is greater than that adhering to actual speech and writing. It is also greater than in the case of the pictorial imagination. While visual imagery makes no register in the external world, the image clearly retains corporeal features. It has a visualized shape and, often, color, which may stand in a pictorial relation to the object imagined. Moreover, this image manifests a quasi-visual permanence that we can inspect with our "mind's eye." Here is a phenomenological basis for Descartes's view that the body is involved in "imagining." However, the auditory speech images used in intellectual thought, by virtue of their arbitrary nature and temporal evanescence appear less bodily in form. As Derrida writes of the inner voice:

> the phenomenological "body" of the signifier seems to fade away at the very moment it is produced; it seems already to belong to the element of ideality. It phenomenologically reduces itself, transforming the worldly opacity of its body into pure diaphaneity.[70]

Moreover, it is not only the body of the signifier, along with one's own body, that disappears in this way, but the body of the referent as well. Via the imagination I picture things that have or could belong to the material world. I envision colors, forms, objects, whose physicality implies that of the imaginer. Yet the referents of abstract thought need not have the same quasi-material presence. For Descartes, such immaterials as God or the soul were primary objects of abstract intellection. Even when dealing with concrete entities, the intellect, he believed, must seek out a conceptual essence unavailable to perception. For Plato it was universal forms such as justice or beauty that were the proper object of rational thought. Whatever one's ontological allegiances— whether one believes in immaterial entities or not—it is clear that such concepts can be manipulated in thought without having a perceptible referent.[71] Yet just as the materiality of a perceptual object correlatively implies that of the perceiver, this disembodied thought-object can seem to imply a disembodied thinker. Rorty refers to this as the paradigm of "the soul as immaterial-because-capable-of-contemplating-univer-sals."[72]

The experience of abstract thought thus provides one of the more powerful derivations for the notion of the rational mind as incorporeal. In this activity, the body of the thinker, the body of the sign, the body of the referent, are all experientially effaced. This strongly encourages the characterization of thought as a disembodied activity engaged in by an immaterial soul.

Margaret Wilson, in her essay, "Cartesian Dualism," searches for the source of Descartes's belief that the understanding can operate independently of the body. She concludes:

> Descartes seems rather surprisingly to have believed that we can reach conclusions about the physical basis or concomitants of the various modes of thought by phenomenological analysis of those modes of thought. The question whether or not the brain is involved in a given mode is connected in Descartes' mind with the question whether the mode of thought somehow involves "corporeal" *imagery.*[73]

I have arrived at similar conclusions. However, I lack Wilson's expressed surprise at the significance of such phenomenologistic concerns. Philosophical doctrines arise out of the life-world and attain popularity and credibility only to the extent that they harmonize with lived experience. In this the Cartesian doctrine is no different; though long criticized by phenomenologists of the lived body, it carries within itself a hidden phenomenology.

To challenge the doctrine of the immaterial intellect, as I have done, need not lead to a naive materialism. The whole doctrine of the lived body, after all, undercuts the conventions of the materialist view. Nor do I wish to deny the possibility of modes of consciousness that transcend those inherent in the human brain. In fact, my personal conviction is that such modes exist. However, to identify transcendent awareness with the exercise of rational thought is, in my belief, a mistake, albeit one prevalent in the Western tradition. Descartes's equating of soul with intellect falsely deifies our cognitive powers and truncates spiritual inquiry. Our interior monologues and abstract rationality are not the stuff of which the sacred is made. Our worship is misplaced if we seek here an immortal and transcendent principle. To challenge the immateriality of this mind is thus hardly a move toward reductionism. On the contrary, it opens up space for new ontologies of body and spirit.

5

The Threatening Body

When man's own experience of himself is seen in a certain way, he perceives the nature of his body as thing-like and soul-moved, which presupposes necessity and dissolves the unity of existence which emerges from the world and results in *forgetting* equally his body and his soul. This occurs when something in *himself strikes* man in such a way that he begins to reflect *upon* himself. . . . As long as we are healthy, nothing strikes us *about* ourselves. However, when our well-being is disturbed, one notices one's own body.

F. J. J. Buytendijk, *Prolegomena to an Anthropological Physiology*

In the previous chapter I have discussed the relationship of the "rational mind" to the phenomenon of bodily disappearance. The tacit nature of certain regions and activities of the body helps support their attribution to an incorporeal mentality. In this chapter, I will discuss the correlative notion of body that arises and its experiential supports.

It is no doubt clear that the Cartesian concept of the body cannot be equated with that which I have been employing throughout this work. I have discussed the lived body as a seat of vitality, action, and thought. Yet precisely to the degree that human capabilities are attributed to an immaterial mind, the notion of "body" must be concomitantly restricted. If reason, for example, is located within an ethereal mind, then the body will be regarded as devoid of higher cognition. It comes to be identified primarily with mindless passions or passive automaticities. Relegated to but one term of a duality, the "body" that remains is but a partial body, defined in terms of a restricted range of abilities.

Moreover, within this duality of which the human being is composed, the body has tended to play the role of secondary or inessential element. For Descartes, as for Plato before him, the true self is often (though not always) identified primarily with the mind or soul.[1] As he writes in *The Discourse,* "this 'me,' that is to say, the soul by which I am what I am, is entirely distinct from body."[2] Conceived of as the locus of subjectivity, it is the soul to which the first-person predicate is applied. "I am a thinking thing," Descartes writes, whereas "I *possess* a body with which I am very intimately conjoined."[3] This scheme reinforces the partiality of the notion of body being employed. Those attributes most definitive of the subject are withheld from corporeality. Body comes to play the role of the Other.

This dualism has not merely an ontological but a valuational dimension. (I will thus refer to this as an "onto-valuational" dualism.) Within the Western philosophical tradition the body has often been regarded as a force of negativity, an obstacle to the soul's attempt to secure knowledge, virtue, or eternal life. This is by no means always the case. For every idealist elevation of sheer mentality, another philosopher awaits to revalue the corporeal sphere. In differing ways this is true of Aristotle in reply to Plato, Marx in reply to Hegel, Merleau-Ponty in reply to Sartre. However, this is precisely a tradition of *reply*. A certain devaluation of the body, either in the form of neglect, deprecation, or outright condemnation, has formed an ongoing theme in our intellectual history to which all those who disagree must begin in response.

This largely negative treatment of the body has by now been frequently commented upon and often regarded as an unfortunate cultural idiosyncrasy. This is indeed somewhat true. Such a distrust of embodiment is by no means a universal phenomenon. To fully understand its ascendency within our culture would necessitate a careful examination of the specific social and historical contexts out of which it developed, including a consideration of salient political, economic, technological, religious, and gender relations.

However, I wish to suggest in this work that our imagery of the body can be understood not only in reference to the cultural projects at play but as an articulation of certain phenomenological possibilities and predispositions arising out of the lived body. Just as the notion of immaterial reason is made possible by the structure of bodily disappearance, the sense of the body as threat is, I will argue, suggested by the phenomenon of dys-appearance. As discussed in chapter 3, the body, forgotten in its seamless functioning, comes to thematic attention particularly at times of breakdown or problematic operation. That the notion of "body" then becomes philosophically associated with dysfunction and Otherness is not a purely contingent matter. Lived experience has already laid the groundwork with its natural bias of attention toward the negative.

I will attempt to make this point in relation to three images of embodiment that have played a central role in the Western tradition. These are, respectively, the body understood as the scene of epistemological error, moral error, and mortality. I will first examine the epistemological framework wherein, as the locus of limited and fallible sense perception, the body has been attacked as a primary source of deception. Next, I will turn to a discourse of morals characterized by a distrust of bodily passions. Finally, I will discuss the medico-theological identification of the body with disease and death. In each case, I will trace out the role played by dys-appearance in encouraging such negativistic portrayals.

This suspicion of embodiment has had a long and variegated history, surfacing, for example, in the Platonism of ancient Greece and Augustinian strains of medieval Christianity, as well as in the works of many other philosophers and periods. A comprehensive survey of this history would lead far beyond the scope of this work. Thus I will continue to use Descartes as a focal example. This may appear more farfetched than his employment in reference to the immateriality of mind. For Descartes seems precisely to remove the body from its historic negative associations. No longer located primarily within the sphere of moral/existential concern, the body is installed within the "neutral" discourse of objective science and metaphysics. It is measurable *res extensa,* not the figure of lust or suffering that dominated previous discussion.

While there is certainly truth here, this interpretation conceals as much as it reveals. The Cartesian project does not so much expunge traditional identifications as transmute and displace them. As I will explore, the body remains for Descartes a place of error, though the emphasis is somewhat shifted from its ethical to its epistemic delusions. Considerations of bodily decay and death form the avowed context of all his work, if not the explicit focus of his texts. While inaugurating the modern concept of the body, Descartes continually relies upon a series of previous Graeco-Christian associations. He is thus valuable both as exemplifying certain long-standing historical themes and as a figure who discloses those twists peculiar to modernity.

Error

Epistemological concerns are at the center of much of the Cartesian project. Descartes inquires as to how we can achieve truth and certainty in our investigations of the world. He finds the answer in the human mind itself. In the *Discourse on Method* and the *Meditations,* Descartes suggests that it is the indubitability of one's own thinking that yields the first certainty on which all other truths must rest. Informed by the "light of nature," able to apprehend clearly and distinctly the existence of God and propositions of logic and mathematics, the mind can then progress to more specific forms of knowledge. In the *Rules for the Direction of the Mind* Descartes had already sketched out the deductive procedures through which we may advance from indubitable propositions to the securing of new truths. It is via the proper use of the rational intellect that truth is revealed and ascertained. And, as has been discussed, that intellect is an immaterial thing.

The body, on the other hand, is conceived of as that which naturally inclines us to error. This is not to say that the body is an unavoidable cause thereof. As a passive machine, devoid of fundamental agency, the body does not have the power to deceive the careful mind. Hence, the direct cause of error is the faculty of will when it exceeds the reach of the understanding.[4] Insofar as the mature mind is trained to suspend decision prior to the achievement of clear and distinct apprehension, error can in all cases be avoided.

Nevertheless, the body constitutes the primary force that clouds the intellect and seduces the will to err. This begins from birth, before the powers of the human mind are developed enough to counter the ill effects of its union with the body:

> Indeed in our early years, our mind was so immersed in the body, that it knew nothing distinctly, although it perceived much sufficiently clearly; and because it even then formed many judgments, numerous prejudices were contracted from which the majority of us can hardly ever hope to become free.[5]

We come to believe through the force of bodily sensations that things outside of us have not only magnitude, figure, and movement, but taste, smell, color, and other such qualities that arise only within the subject. In *The Principles of Philosophy,* Descartes labels this childhood prejudice the principal cause of error, noting that it continues to exert its power even after we reach the age of maturity.[6] Moreover, as a result of its corporeal associations, the mind finds it extremely difficult to engage in intellection purified of the senses or imagination.[7] The consequence is further deception; we not only misconstrue the nature of material objects but tend to disbelieve in the existence of immaterials.

Thus, according to Descartes, the human will and intellect are always engaged in a rearguard action against an ever present deceiver. Mistakes are not so much a matter of the mind positively choosing to err as failing to undo the distortions that the body has introduced. To uncover truth is to forcibly bring this body to heel:

> I shall now close my eyes, I shall stop my ears, I shall call away all my senses, I shall efface even from my thoughts all the images of corporeal things, or at least (for that is hardly possible) I shall esteem them as vain and false.[8]

It is true that by the end of the *Meditations,* Descartes recognizes a certain circumscribed validity to bodily perceptions. Because God is fundamentally nondeceptive, Descartes is sure that the perceived world is not a complete illusion and external bodies do exist. Moreover, he has reached assurance that "my senses more frequently indicate to me truth than falsehood respecting the things which concern that which is beneficial to the body."[9] Sense perceptions were placed within us to signify what is useful or harmful to us as composite beings and are mostly reliable within this pragmatic context.[10] However, in relation to the truth that principally interests Descartes, that is, scientific truth concerning the essence of external objects, "they can teach me nothing but what is most obscure and confused."[11] As did Plato before him, Descartes refers to the body as a "prison"[12] within this epistemological context, that which exerts "an obstructive effect on the soul . . . always a hindrance to the mind in its thinking."[13]

Error and Dys-appearance

If I seek to know what time of day it is I gauge the light outside my window or glance at a clock. How many people are in the room? I look around. What kind of plant have we here? I gaze at it, smell, touch it, turn it to examine the underside. On the face of it, it would seem that my body and its sensorimotor powers constitute the principal means whereby I know the world.

Why then does Descartes focus upon the body as a place of epistemological obstruction? This cannot be understood without reference to developments in early modern science. The Copernican assertion that the earth goes around the sun had reversed the naive testimony of the senses and replaced their authority with that of mathematics. The power of mathematics to reveal truth unavailable to immediate perception was further confirmed by the work of Galileo and Kepler. It is within this ambience that Descartes comes to regard material reality as *res extensa,* a substance wholly reducible to its geometrical properties. If this is true, the panoply of colors, smells, tastes, and sounds revealed by our body is a shadow dance, a seductive deception.

Many works have focused on these historical roots of Cartesianism.[14] However, such historical developments can only bring to the fore, intensify, or diminish possibilities latent in the lived body itself. I wish to investigate those structures of embodiment which render possible and give experiential support to the Cartesian view. Primary among these is the operation of dys-appearance; we are made aware of our body precisely at times of dysfunction. As I will try to show, such dysfunctional moments inaugurate and channel Cartesian reflection on the body.

To make this point I will turn to Descartes's own account of those events which led to his philosophical reading of the body. The *Medita-*

tions, if its structure is taken seriously, is not just a work of logical argumentation but provides a rich phenomenology of personal experience. In the *Sixth Meditation,* Descartes informs us that initially he naively trusted what his body told him:

> But afterwards many experiences little by little destroyed all the faith which I had rested in my senses; for I from time to time observed that those towers which from afar appeared to me to be round, more closely observed seemed square, and that colossal statues raised on the summit of these towers, appeared as quite tiny statues when viewed from the bottom; and so in an infinitude of other cases I found error in judgments founded on the external senses.[15]

It is helpful to examine the phenomenological structure of such occurrences. Ordinarily, as I move through the world there is a seamless continuity of my perspectives; I see constant objects through a variety of shifting perceptual profiles. I need not thematize the intricate spatiotemporal synthesis my body accomplishes at each moment. It is the taken-for-granted that enables me to focus outward. The body is still taken for granted by Descartes in the prephilosophical stage that corresponds to such experiences. However, reflection on embodiment is compelled by the moment of dys-appearance when the body is away, apart, from its own previous states or norms of ordinary functioning. In chapter 3, I discussed the self-divergence involved in vital disturbances such as pain and illness. Yet here it is precisely one's body *as perceiver* that diverges from its own previous state. Descartes's present perspective reveals the illusory nature of what he earlier thought he saw, e.g., the square tower that first appeared round. This problematic divergence, calling into question corporeal functioning, drives one to reflect back upon the body.

Continuing his discussion of those experiences which first destroyed his perceptual faith, Descartes notes that he had found error:

> not only in those [judgments] founded on the external senses, but even in those founded on the internal as well; for is there anything more intimate or more internal than pain? And yet I have learned from some persons whose arms or legs have been cut off, that they sometimes seemed to feel pain in the part which had been amputated, which made me think that I could not be quite certain that it was a certain member which pained me, even although I felt pain in it.[16]

We see dys-appearance again at work in forcing the body before our view. In the case of the phantom limb patient, the body is literally disrupted, dismembered in fact. Moreover, this physical disruption inaugurates an even deeper set of phenomenological divergences. The coenesthetic experiences of a still-present limb differ from the evidences of amputation offered up by all the other senses. The habitual corporeal schema struggles with its novel, altered form. The inner experience of the patient conflicts with what all others see from without. This body becomes a field of spatial, temporal, functional, and intersubjective ruptures that lead inevitably to its thematization.

The body most comes into view at such times of disruption, presenting itself as a problem to be solved, whether on the plane of ordinary experience or philosophical reflection. This principle is etched on the Cartesian corpus—everywhere are disrupted bodies. For example, the *Meditations* commences with two more such bodies, that of the dreamer and that of the madman. In the former case, a problematic divergence exists between one's own corporeal states. Upon awakening one sees the illusory nature of all that was apprehended by the body asleep. One is led to reflect upon corporeality: "I am awake now and then I was dreaming." In the case of the madman it is an intersubjective rupture that brings the body to the fore. There is a divergence between what the sane person and the madman perceive, which calls into question the very conditions of perception. Descartes is thus led to reflect on the "violent vapors of black bile" coursing through the madman's cerebellum.[17]

Moreover, Descartes is struck by the ability of bodily disturbances not only to give rise to error but to cripple the very search for truth. As mentioned earlier, for Descartes the soul proceeds with intellectual thought entirely free from the body. Yet he cannot help but note the ability of body to hinder thought in situations of pain and fatigue[18] or via "the bad disposition of the bodily organs."[19] In such cases of dysappearance, a corporeal presence thrusts itself undeniably into awareness. He concludes that the rational soul is simply unable to disassociate itself from "a brain which is too soft or damp, as in children, or otherwise ill tempered, as in those who are lethargic, apoplectic, or frenetic, or as in all of us when we are deeply asleep."[20] The soul can only detach itself from a certain sort of body, one calm, healthy, and awake.

This Cartesian epistemology might be termed a *motivated misreading*. That is, his conclusions are motivated by lived experience, albeit as misread into a reified ontology. The body draws his philosophical attention particularly at times of perceptual error, injury, madness, disease, fatigue, excessive passion, and pain. For it is at such times that the body opacifies, clearly exhibiting its role in experience. This skew of attention then encourages a dualist reading. For when dysfunctioning, the body seems most Other to the self, a force opposed to the understanding and will. Moreover, this alien body surfaces as something negative and dis-valued. Onto-valuational dualism captures in a conceptual system what is first suggested by immediate experience.

Moreover, as discussed in chapter 3, it is these disruptive moments, not those times of unproblematic operation, that demand hermeneutic and practical strategies of repair. This further focuses attention on the dysfunctional. The delusions and limitations of the body must be iso-lated, studied, traced to their source, in order to facilitate practices of control. These failings thus become the center of discourse. Descartes thus gives disproportionate attention to diseased and deceptive bodies compared to his brief treatment of the positive.

This tendency toward a negative epistemics established by dys-appearance is reinforced by the complementary operation of bodily dis-appearance. While the body is highlighted in deceptive modes, it tends to be taken for granted at times of accurate perception. The revelatory power of the body rests precisely upon its self-effacement. Moreover, as has been discussed, this self-effacement is most marked in the case of abstract thought. Insofar as such thinking is regarded as the royal road to truth, this road seems to lead away from the body. When the body reclaims attention it is in the guise of an obstacle on the path: for exam-ple, the pain or fatigue that interferes with thought. Thus, for Des-cartes, as for Plato before him, a "disembodied" state is highly to be valued.

While experientially motivated, this interpretation remains a mis-reading. The body cannot be identified primarily with its episodes of dys-appearance and exiled from the domain of truth. We are reminded of the body at times of hindrance only because a rupture has occurred in a more general, though tacit, context of operation: the body as the means whereby world is disclosed. In fact, this general context is im-plicitly present within Descartes's examples, deconstructing his partial-ized epistemology from within. That is, each example of corporeal error is exposed precisely by the corrective action of the body. Descartes dis-covers his mistake regarding the shape of a tower only because his new, closer view reveals the truth. The error of the phantom limb patient, fooled by coenesthesias, is exposed by all the other senses combined. We know the falsity of the madman's perceptions by virtue of our own con-sensually-validated sight. It is when the truth of our surroundings floods in upon awakening that we realize the deceptive nature of our dreams. As Merleau-Ponty writes:

> when an illusion dissipates, when an appearance suddenly breaks up, it is
> always for the profit of a new appearance which takes up again for its

own account the ontological function of the first. . . . The dis-illusion is
the loss of one evidence only because it is the acquisition of *another evidence*.[21]

The experience of corporeal deception is possible only because the lived
body, through its perceptual and symbolic powers, is an open horizon of
further disclosure and truth. It is this wider context of embodiment as
the place of knowledge that rests unacknowledged in the margins of the
text.

This is no less true of the cultural context in which Descartes dwelled.
One might refer, for example, to the Copernican rejection of Ptolemaic
astronomy as inaugurating an episode of cultural dys-appearance. Attention came to be focused on the body-as-deceptive when it was realized
that naive perception could so mislead. The sun does not go around the
earth despite the testimony of our senses. Yet even here it is the embodied
subject, not a purified mind, that corrects prior falsity. Admittedly, the
fathers of modernity turned to mathematical science, not the senses, for
truth. But as thinkers such as Husserl,[22] Merleau-Ponty,[23] Kuhn,[24] and
Heelan[25] have pointed out, science and mathematics have their own embodied roots in modes of measurement, perception, and instrumentation. Our body is not left behind in such "higher-level" pursuits. Rather its
powers are extended and sublimated through the use of technologies, the
rigor of experimental technique, and the restructuring of perception by
novel paradigms.

Moral Error

My discussion of bodily error would be incomplete if confined to the
epistemological realm. For Descartes is also concerned to account for
and remedy *moral* error. As his moral psychology is far less developed
than his epistemology and metaphysics I will give this topic briefer
treatment. However, it opens a door to a theme of great import: the moral condemnation of the body. In the Western tradition, particularly as
shaped by Platonism and Christianity, there has been an abiding distrust of bodily passions and desires. Here too, I will suggest, the phenomenon of dys-appearance plays its formative role.

It is in *The Passions of the Soul* that Descartes systematically addresses
the place of the body vis-à-vis the good life. For a "passion" of the soul,
in Descartes's primary usage, is a feeling or emotion principally caused,
maintained, and fortified by the body.[26] Descartes's moral characterization of the passions closely parallels his epistemology of the senses. Just
as sense perceptions yield a certain pragmatic truth concerning what is
beneficial to us as embodied beings, so do the passions:

their natural use is to incite the soul to consent and contribute to the actions which may serve to maintain the body, or to render it in some manner more perfect.[27]

However, as with the senses, this natural utility comes hand in hand with a tendency to deceive. First, there are many things hurtful to the body that cause no sadness or even produce joy, and conversely, many beneficial things that seem to us distasteful.[28] Thus, the passions may lead us to act against our better interests. Second, even if they are properly aligned, the passions still mislead via their power of exaggeration:

> they almost always cause the good things, as well as the evil, to seem much greater and more important than they are; so that they incite us to seek after the one and flee from the others with more ardour and care than is desirable.[29]

Finally, corporeal passions tend to involve fleeting pleasures and pains, not the more durable goods of the soul.[30] For all such reasons, the prism of body-based emotion distorts the true nature and import of objects in our life. The body leads us astray regarding how best to live, just as it does concerning scientific truth.

Thus, in the ethical no less than the epistemological sphere, Descartes searches for pragmatic strategies to overcome a problematic body. As he recognizes, one cannot simply will away a passion given its strong physical base.[31] However, just as one can suspend judgment vis-à-vis the senses until proper understanding is reached, so action can be suspended in the face of strong emotion. He advises restraint until the initial passion has quieted,[32] or we have carefully considered reasons that oppose our bias.[33] Eventually, through reflection on counterarguments and examples one can even change one's emotions themselves.[34] Through such mechanisms, "there is no soul so feeble that it cannot, if well directed, acquire an absolute power over its passions."[35]

Descartes was not an antiemotionalist or as extreme as certain of his religious predecessors. He regards the passions as "all good in their nature," insofar as evil uses and excesses are avoided.[36] Many are pleasurable, can incite within us positive thoughts, and even act to fortify our virtues.[37] However, this proper utility is realized only under the direction and mastery of the soul. Reason must continually monitor the reactive tendencies to which the body is heir and counteract its deceptive pulls. Virtue thus involves "a firm and constant resolution to carry out whatever reason recommends without being diverted by passion or appetite."[38] The body is again entrapped primarily within a negative discourse.

DYS-APPEARANCE AND THE PASSIONS

To understand one experiential source for this moral distrust of body, I will briefly turn to the corporeal structure of emotion. I have previously discussed the notion of the *microchiasm* in relation to the brain; this organ constitutes an anatomical intertwining of surface and depth, sensorimotor and visceral characteristics, recapitulating the chiasmatic structure of the body at large. The same is true of the emotions on a functional level. On the one hand, they are an aspect of our ecstatic relatedness to world. We always experience our environment through a particular mood.[39] The world is perceived very differently depending on whether one is overjoyed or depressed. Moreover, emotion inaugurates our motor projects, propelling us toward desired goals.[40]* This is reflected in the common etymological root shared by the words *motion* and *emotion*. Yet, while guiding our sensorimotor engagements, emotionality is also rooted in the visceral. Our passions often relate directly or indirectly to visceral needs for food, warmth, sexuality, rest, etc. Moreover, it is in the secretion of hormones, the realignment of visceral processes, that strong emotions find their register. For example, fear, like rage, relies on a glandular flood of adrenaline and the increased sympathetic tone of the autonomic nervous system, transforming patterns of blood flow, body temperature, cardiac and respiratory function. As Descartes notes, such physical changes predispose not only the body but the soul itself for flight.[41] That is, our visceral states help shape our perceptions and desires.

As I earlier discussed, the visceral body always recedes to a certain degree from the personal will. The visceral exhibits an "I must" and "I cannot"; I am compelled by organic needs and functions in a manner over which I have no direct control. This is one source, though not the only one, of the passivity of soul captured in the term "passion." As Descartes recounts, once an emotion holds sway I cannot simply will it away. I cannot, for example, shut off an adrenaline-charged fear in the same way in which I can shut my eyes. Descartes thus counsels indirect strategies of delay, restraint, imagery, and self-persuasion. As discussed in chapter 2, the relations of personalized to visceral self are always characterized by such indirection.

Hence, our emotional life exhibits certain aspects of depth disappearance, that mode of absence characteristic of the visceral. In this case, depth disappearance is manifested specifically in the area of control; the emotions, at least for most of us, escape to a degree from our willful command. The same is true of passionate desires, such as those of a sexual nature. Sexuality too is a microchiasm: while a mode of sensori-motor relation to the world, it exhibits a visceral autonomy. The arising of desire and its enactment in complex physiological changes including lubrication, erection, orgasm, and ejaculation, are never fully under the control of the egoic self. As Augustine laments of lust:

> Sometimes the impulse is an unwanted intruder, sometimes it abandons the eager lover, and desire cools off in the body while it is at boiling heat in the mind.[42]

This depth disappearance of emotions and desires can lead in turn to dys-appearance.[43]* Somewhat involuntary in nature, our passions can surface as a disruptive force hindering our projects. Lust can over-whelm our intellectual commitments and moral scruples. We may be paralyzed by fear or consumed by an unwanted anger. Just as the body is remembered when pain or sickness interferes with our intentions, so too when powerful passions rebel. At such times the body dys-appears, surfacing as an alien or threatening thing. For Augustine, this re-belliousness represents a physical imprint of original sin; in punishment for Adam's disobedience to God, God implanted lust within us, render-ing our flesh disobedient to our will.[44]

It is not only the visceral dimension of passion but the complexity of human appetition in general that gives rise to dys-appearance. Cravings of one sort may battle with those that pull us in an opposite direction. Passions of the moment can conflict with long-term goods. As such, the desiring body can begin to crumble and self-diverge, as does the organic body in illness. We thematize the body at such problematic times in a way we need not do when we are unified.

Descartes's moral discourse no less than his epistemology is shaped by this attentional skew. While acknowledging the salutary nature of much of our passionate life, Descartes focuses upon ways of understand-ing and overcoming its moments of hindrance. It is these moments, not times when the body is tacit and ego-congruent, that demand attention, interpretation, and control. This is reflected in the very genesis of *The Passions of the Soul;* Descartes's text grew out of a correspondence with Elizabeth, who, driven by emotional distress and poor health, inquired as to how mastery of the passions could be achieved.[45]

To clarify this phenomenological point, I will focus upon the example of fear. In preparing for a challenge, I may find myself overcome by this contrary emotion. Prior to its advent I have no need to thematize the body. Consideration of my obligations is undertaken in a calm and rational fashion. At such times no strong bodily agitations, no racing pulse, or

heaving heart forces the body before my view. Herein lies another phenomenological motivation, to be added to those in the previous chapter,
for the Platonic-Cartesian sense of rationality as disembodied. In that
relatively emotionless state considered most characteristic of "reason,"
the body experientially disappears.

Moreover, the body disappears insofar as it remains aligned with my
egoic will. That is, before the onset of fear I am more or less able to take
my body for granted. It is that from which I will actualize my goals
without the need of explicit self-reflection or self-control. The virtuous,
the compliant body calls for no particular attention.

This is no longer the case when fear erupts, throwing an obstacle in
the path of my will. A physicality that moments before was invisible
now asserts itself via sweating palms, a nervous twitch, a choking voice,
an almost irresistible urge to run. Though it is congruent with my overall values and long-term interests to press on, my body, as it were, has
another idea. It emerges as away, apart, from my desired state and from
my experienced sense of self.

Such phenomena thus lend their support to onto-valuational dualism. That is, they can be schematized, as they are by Descartes, as a
battle between the soul and the recalcitrant body. Descartes rejects the
notion that the soul wars with itself, for it "has not in itself any diversity
of parts."[46] Rather, it is "the body, to which alone we must attribute
every thing which can be observed in us that is opposed to our reason."
He pictures the pineal gland as the site of strife, "thrust to one side by
the soul, and to the other by the animal spirits." An experiential sense of
inner division is thus translated into metaphysical dualism.[47*]

Death

In addition to its treatment within the contexts of epistemology and
ethics, Descartes also addresses the body as the biological/existential
scene of life. That is, the body constitutes the precondition of human
vitality, the place of youth and aging, health and illness. Yet just as the
body is associated with hindrance vis-à-vis knowledge and right action,
so too within this vital realm. Largely taken for granted as the place of
life, well-being, and growth, Descartes addresses the body as the scene
of decay, disease, and most especially, death.

Indeed, I will suggest that the figure of the mortal body is not only a
crucial motivator of Descartes's work but central to his methodology
and metaphysics. Only with this recognition will the full significance of
dys-appearance emerge.

Descartes's Motivation

I will begin by examining those considerations which, according to Descartes, impelled his far-reaching quest for knowledge. In Descartes's prefatory note to the *Meditations,* he presents this study as having two major goals. The first is to provide proof of God's existence, while the second involves introducing philosophical grounds for the belief "that the human soul does not perish with the body."[48] Descartes's famous proof of the distinctness of mind and body is meant to stand in service to the latter goal. As he wrote in the earlier *Discourse on Method:*

> As a matter of fact, when one comes to know how greatly they differ, we understand much better the reasons which go to prove that our soul is in its nature entirely independent of body, and in consequence that it is not liable to die with it. And then, inasmuch as we observe no other causes capable of destroying it, we are naturally inclined to judge that it is immortal.[49]

In a letter to Huygens, Descartes makes clear that this proof held a personal significance. While asserting the belief that souls outlast their bodies and pass on to a "sweeter and more tranquil life," he confesses that theological teachings alone fail to persuade. He, like most men, needs the testimony of natural reasons.[50]

Thus, Descartes's metaphysical explorations are partially motivated by the existential threat posed by the perishable body. The *Meditations* is a text inaugurated not only by a confrontation with error but with death.[51] Some have argued that Descartes's avowed interest in theological matters, such as the immortality of the soul, was but a smokescreen designed to permit his scientific investigations to proceed unhampered by the Church. I am not in agreement with such a position. Biographical material, such as the above letter to Huygens, suggests the sincerity of his concerns. However, even if such a position were true it would not undermine the point at hand. For a preoccupation with the body as diseased and dying is central to Descartes's scientific projects as well.

Descartes concludes the *Discourse on Method* by laying out the program of his future work:

> But I will just say that I have resolved not to employ the time which remains to me in life in any other matter than in endeavouring to acquire some knowledge of nature, which shall be of such a kind that it will enable us to arrive at rules for Medicine more assured than those which have as yet been attained.[52]

Descartes argues that the preservation of health is in fact the governing aim of scientific investigation, because health is "the chief blessing and the foundation of all other blessings in this life."[53] While maintaining a rather low opinion of the medicine of his day, he is sanguine about the results a true science could yield. We could be freed from "an infinitude of maladies" and possibly of the "infirmities of age" through the proper knowledge of causes and treatments.[54] Though at various points in his career, Descartes concedes that he was far from bringing such ends to fruition,[55] he never abandoned his therapeutic goal. Some ten years after the writing of the *Discourse* he reasserts that "the preservation of health has always been the principal end of my studies."[56] It is with reference to this project that he begins the *Description of the Human Body,* on which he was at work shortly before his death.[57]

Once again, biographical material bears testimony to the personal nature of Descartes's concern. A sickly youth, condemned by doctors to die young,[58] Descartes sought in later life to postpone death beyond what was considered humanly possible. In 1637 he writes to Huygens:

> The fact that my hair is turning gray warns me that I should spend all my time trying to set back the process. That is what I am working on now, and I hope my efforts will succeed even though I lack sufficient experimentation.[59]

In later letters he expresses hopes of living to more than a hundred years through maintaining proper habits, taking great pains to protect his health, and utilizing his medical knowledge.[60] Ultimately, all such efforts did not prevent a fatal encounter with pneumonia. This was even something of a joke at the time; a Belgian newspaper reported, "In Sweden a fool has just died who used to say that he could live as long as he wanted."[61] If his medical studies were of little avail in postponing death, his metaphysics may at least have provided the assurance that he sought. Clerselier recounts how, two days before he died, wracked with fever and convinced the end was near, Descartes spoke thusly: "My soul, you have been a captive for a long time; now the hour has come when you must leave your prison, this body; you must bear this separation with joy and courage."[62]

Thus it is possible to discover a hidden unity of motivation between Descartes's metaphysical and scientific investigations: that is, the threat posed by sickness and death. The dualism of the *Meditations* provides Descartes with a two-sided response. In proving that the body is a mechanical, mathematical entity, free of all soul attributes, he lays the groundwork for a modern scientific medicine. In this way he hopes to discover ways to indefinitely prolong embodied life. But such a life cannot go on forever. Hence, the necessity of proving the immaterial nature of the rational soul, and thereby its immortality. Body and soul, science and theology: Descartes's schema serves to combat death on all fronts.

Mortality and Dys-appearance

In this way, dys-appearance again plays a role in provoking Cartesian discourse. As the place of health and life, embodiment can be forgotten. Viscerality sustains us according to the tacit "it can," while the sensorimotor self is directed ecstatically toward its world of involvements. The body-as-living generally functions as the horizon within which everything else is disclosed, not as an object of scrutiny. Yet when illness or mortality loom before us, this body is brought into sharp relief. As discussed in chapter 3, one is seized in an immediate way by physical pain and dysfunction. Moreover, the body can dys-appear not only as the scene of actual but potential disruption. Descartes's grey hairs, foretelling his mortality, are enough to stimulate redoubled investigations. Though none of us has ever experienced our death, it ever seeds our body, waiting to blossom. It is foretold from within by episodes of pain, injury, and illness, by the body's gradual changes and loss of function with age. And in death lies the ultimate mode of dys-appearance. The body in its aspect as that-which-must-die can constitute a threat to all of one's goals. It can sever or transform all relations, bring all projects to a halt, threaten one's very existence as an "I." This body thus emerges as an ego-alien force that demands thematization. That is not to say that one cannot come to terms with death or even affirm it. Yet this is always the result of an interpretive process and often a profound existential struggle. The body-as-mortal poses a core problematic that cries out for hermeneutic and pragmatic therapies.

Descartes's scientific and metaphysical work is just such a therapy. He seeks a way to overcome bodily illness and aging and to prove that death cannot capture the soul. Just as he sought a treatment for the deceptiveness of the senses and the passions, so for the body's fragility. In all three cases, the human intellect not only discovers the solution but finds that it itself, *is* the solution. It is intellectual reason that overcomes sense deception and masters the pull of the passions. Similarly, it is reason that forms the core of the soul destined to outlive the perishable body. Descartes here valorizes reason in a metaphysical-theological mode, hearkening back to the Platonic tradition. Yet Descartes also inaugurates a modern age where reason is valorized in a scientific, technological form. It becomes the instrument for conquering nature, expunging disease, vastly increasing the human lifespan. This mode of transcendence employs moves that draw upon but also transform earlier

discursive strategies. In order to explore this point I will turn my attention from Descartes's motivation to his scientific methodology and
correlative metaphysics. Here too can be found the hidden operation of
disease, death, and dys-appearance.

Descartes's Method and Metaphysics

In the *Meditations* Descartes supports his theory of pineal gland mind-
body interactionism via evidence provided by phantom limb amputees,
dropsy victims, the cerebrally disordered, sufferers of sensory loss and
referred pain.[63] This illustrates what I would term the *analytic* role of
dys-appearance. The tacit synergy of the bodily field conceals the operation of individual parts and organs. Yet this synergy is what injury and
disease disrupt, performing a natural analytic function. The dysfunctioning body first stands out as separate from its world; similarly,
discrete mechanisms stand out from the body gestalt by virtue of their
particular dysfunctions. Hence, the modern scientist still studies normal physiology through experimental lesions, the information provided
by disease states, and the disruptions created by artificial laboratory conditions. The normal is understood via the pathological, for therein the
body is made to dys-appear.[64*]

For Descartes, clues gathered from the body discomforted and diseased were assimilated to a general knowledge structure resting upon
the body as dead. At certain periods, Descartes had a habit of almost
daily visits to butcher shops, engaging in a careful examination and dissection of animal organs.[65] Such work continued for at least eleven
years, informing the large section of Descartes's corpus involved with
medical physiology: *The Treatise of Man, Description of the Human Body,
The Passions of the Soul, Dioptrics,* as well as a significant section of the
Discourse on Method.

One's methodology of investigation is inevitably intertwined with
one's model of the real; a certain manner of questioning the world supports and solidifies a particular worldview, just as a worldview suggests
the research strategies to be employed. Hence, Descartes's extensive uti-
lization of dissection implies a central role for death in his metaphysics
of embodiment.

The antecedent for this is already to be found in historical associations of the living body with death. Plato refers to the Orphic equation
of *soma* and *sema*—the body thought of as a tomb for the soul.[66] For
Augustine, as for many other medieval thinkers, the body, when taken
strictly by itself, is understood as something devoid of animation, psychological predicates, or feeling.[67] Only soul provides the infusion of
life; the body alone is something like a corpse.

On the surface, Descartes seems to make a radical break with this tradition. Reconceiving the soul as intellectual mind, he explicitly disassociates it from the animal or vegetative life-soul of the ancients.[68] He regards the body's own mechanical processes as the cause of physiological vitality. As Descartes writes to Henry More, "I do not deny life to animals, since I regard it as consisting simply in the heat of the heart."[69] Nor is the cessation of life caused by the departure of soul:

> death never comes to pass by reason of the soul, but only because some one of the principal parts of the body decays: and we may judge that the body of a living man differs from that of a dead man just as does a watch or other automaton (i.e. a machine that moves of itself), when it is wound up and contains in itself the corporeal principle of those movements for which it is designed along with all that is requisite for its action, from the same watch or other machine when it is broken and when the principle of its movement ceases to act.[70]

Descartes thus defies custom by locating the principle of life directly in the body, not the soul. Yet, what appears a reversal of tradition is in fact but a transmutation. For this concession of life to the body is only made possible by a deeper concession to death. As the above quote indicates, the body's so-called life is modeled according to the workings of an inanimate machine. The body can constitute the place of life only because life itself has been fundamentally reconceived according to the lifeless. As Descartes concludes the *Treatise of Man,* "the fire which burns continually in its heart . . . is of no other nature than all those fires that occur in inanimate bodies."[71] Without the soul's presence, the body would remain an operative machine, but one devoid of any truly experiential life. Dissection of the corpse can provide a method of studying the live body only because the latter is itself a sort of animated corpse.[72]*

Moreover, this image of embodiment closely relates to Descartes's overarching ontology of the physical world. As Carolyn Merchant discusses, mechanism effects something like "the death of nature."[73] The Aristotelian ascription of telos to the natural world and the neo-Platonic attribution of occult sympathies and antipathies are equally expunged by the Cartesian worldview. No longer is nature conceived of as fundamentally subjective and alive. It is simply *res extensa,* a plenum of passive matter moved by the operation of mechanical forces. The human soul is a small corner of experience dwelling within this vast inanimate universe. The modeling of the human body on the corpse is part and parcel of this larger shift to the primacy of the lifeless within modern cosmology.

Hans Jonas has argued an important and intriguing thesis: that the corpse actually played a central role in inaugurating mechanism's ontology of death. For animism dominated earlier conceptions of nature; life abounds in our immediate province with plants, animals, earth, wind, and water all in motion and seemingly saturated with psyche. Only the phenomenon of death poses an ongoing challenge to this ontology of life.

> The "unto dust shalt thou return" which every corpse calls out to the living, the finality of the state which its decay opposes to the transience of life, must have first and ever again forced "matter" as bare and lifeless into the reluctant human view, and it never ceased to renew the challenge which panvitalist creed, in the funeral cult, could appease but not silence. Whether and when this contradiction came to a crisis depended on historical circumstances with which the "death" motif had to ally itself so that at some time it could overwhelm the "life motif." But when this happened, the naive monism broke up into a dualism, with whose growth the traits of the bewildering sight from which it had started— the sight of the corpse—could progressively spread over the face of the physical All. Death in fact conquered external reality.[74]

In my terms, the body-in-death dys-appears as something alien. The corpse is no longer the instrument of subjectivity but lies inert, recalcitrant, the very model of passivity and opposition. It becomes emblematic of a different order of being. To understand the experiences that help give rise to Cartesian dualism, it is thus necessary to turn to a phenomenology of the corpse.

The Corpse

As previously mentioned, my own corpse is experienced in an anticipatory fashion, residing implicitly within my living body. Exhaustion reminds me of the sheer weight of my limbs; an X ray reveals my skeleton to vision; accidents remind me of my exquisite vulnerability; in aging, I perceive the loss of faculties and skills. These reminders of death constitute a force of dys-appearance, recalling me to my embodied state. The corpse is always approaching from within.

However, it is also that which never arrives. Where I am as a living, experiencing body, the corpse is not, and vice versa. Though I can imagine what I will look like in my coffin, this is not a sight I can see with my eyes. As such, the body-as-dead partakes of certain aspects of depth disappearance; that is, it necessarily withdraws from the egoic self. Specifically, the corpse exhibits a temporal mode of depth disappearance, as do the sleeping and prenatal body previously discussed. The association of death with sleep found in the art and mythology of many cultures expresses this phenomenological commonality; both bodies withdraw from sensorimotor engagement with the world. And just as the embryonic body always precedes the advent of one's vision, so the corpse always follows its departure. The corpse is the temporal mode of depth disappearance belonging to the future, a constantly approaching future that yet ever recedes, a necessary terminus at which the "I" cannot arrive.

Thus Socrates, when asked by Crito how he wishes to be buried, laughs at this paradoxical question.

> He thinks that I am the one whom he will see presently lying dead, and he asks how he is to bury me! . . . . you must assure him that when I am dead I shall not stay, but depart and be gone. That will help Crito to bear it more easily, and keep him from being distressed on my account when he sees my body being burned or buried, as if something dreadful were happening to me, or from saying at the funeral that it is Socrates whom he is laying out or carrying to the grave or burying.[75]

When the corpse is there, Socrates is not. A meditation on this corpse approaching from within inaugurates and orients the *Phaedo*.

Yet this is not the primary figure of the corpse operative in Cartesian method. For Descartes it is the corpse as object of dissection that provides the key to scientific knowledge. That is, while Socrates refers to his *own* corpse in the anticipatory mode, Descartes dwells upon the actualized corpse of the *Other*.

In this shift of perspective is found a clue to the modernist transmutation Descartes effects. The body has often been associated with disease, decay, and death from ancient to contemporary times. Yet for the Greeks and medievals this was a concern articulated primarily from the first-person perspective. There was an existential preoccupation with one's own finitude as mortal being. It is the death of the subject that was of concern. As has been discussed, this personal preoccupation with mortality is a motivating factor in Descartes's work. Yet his strategy for overcoming this first-person threat is precisely to capture the body fully in the third person. It is the body of the Other that Descartes anatomizes, his own body then reconstructed on such a model. As he writes in the *Meditations*:

> In the first place, then, I considered myself as having a face, hands, arms, and all that system of members composed of bones and flesh *as seen in a corpse* which I designated by the name of body.[76]

The corpse from the third-person point of view is the phenomenological opposite of that as viewed from the first person. Whereas my corpse is wrapped in an ineluctable absence, a withdrawal from self-experience, the corpse of the Other thrusts itself into my view. There is a dys-appearance that renders all perspicuous. The Other's viscera, hidden within bodily depths during life, can now be opened up and explored. Depth disappearance is all but eradicated. So too is surface disappearance overcome. That is, ordinarily I do not thematize the Other's body per se; we exist in a cosubjectivity, directed outward to a common world. But death is precisely what severs (or renders problematic) this cosubjectivity, inaugurating the objectified relation. Whereas yesterday I cavorted with a living person, today I confront the physicality of the corpse. It lies there, strangely unmoving, unseeing flesh, no longer a play of absence and reference. Body qua body now emerges, freezing my gaze within its boundaries as the lived body never could.[77*]

This figure of the third-person corpse has profoundly influenced the modern understanding of the body, coexisting uneasily with and in certain cases supplanting other ways of approaching embodiment. I will briefly illustrate this point in relation to modern medicine.

THE CORPSE AND MODERN MEDICINE

Descartes's reliance upon dissection exemplifies the epistemological power of dys-appearance. We can inspect a dead body in a way we cannot the living. Modern medicine, profoundly Cartesian in spirit, has continued to use the corpse as a methodological tool and a regulative ideal. Medical education begins with the cadaver, just as the clinical case ends with the pathoanatomical dissection. Death unveils the truths of the inner body and its diseases. As Foucault[78] and Engelhardt[79] describe, this visceral revelation has served to reorganize medical understanding as a whole. That is, in the beginning of the nineteenth century, classifications of disease shifted from a basis in the experienced symptoms of the patient to a system of definition according to the organic lesions found at death. Pathoanatomical findings were progressively regarded as more foundational and real than "epiphenomenal" symptoms. The growth of medical technology, another defining feature of modern medicine, was stimulated by this conceptual shift. Reiser recounts how doctors sought a variety of instruments that would allow direct perception of the living viscera just as dissection exposed them in the corpse. A nineteenth-century physician thus extols the merits of the stethoscope: "We anatomize by auscultation (if I may say so), while the patient is yet alive."[80]

Along with this overcoming of depth disappearance, an eradication of surface disappearance is constituitive of the modern medico-scientific ideal. While the body remains a living ecstasis it is never fully caught in the web of causal explanation. I may attempt to understand the movements of another by tracking internal chains of physiological events. Yet the lived body is that which always projects beyond such a perspective. Its movements are responses to a perceived world and a desired future, born of meaning, not just mechanical impingements. This bodily ecstasis constitutes an absence that undermines attempts to analyze the body and to predict and control its responses. Only the corpse seems to render such a project triumphant. The dead body is at last self-contained. It is a sheerly material and predictable thing.

Truth, understood in Heideggerian terms, is a process of simultaneous revealing-concealing. Aspects of world are disclosed only by virtue of obscuring others. While the epistemic revelation inherent in the dys-appearing corpse has subserved the powerful accomplishments of medical science, it has also brought about a kind of concealment. Key distortions are inevitably introduced when the dead body is taken as model for the living. This, I will now suggest, is one source of the reductionist and objectivist tendencies of modern Cartesian medicine.

As noted above, the lived body operates according to gestalt relations, each organ cooperating with one another, the senses synesthetically intertwining, movement permeating perception. Yet a reductionist rather than syncretic model of the body will be encouraged when the corpse becomes paradigmatic. For in death all the linkages of the lived body are disrupted. The body dissolves from an operational whole into discrete organs and tissues, which can be studied in isolation. This then fosters an atomistic concept of disease and therapeutic response. Such can be seen, for example, in the trend toward medical specialization, with a different practitioner for each individual organ.

Moreover, notions of embodiment based upon the corpse can lead to an objectivist, depersonalized medicine. The physician need not attend to the patient's intentionality when he or she is conceived of as physiological machine. As Merchant speaks of the "death of nature," here one might speak of the "death of the patient." Diagnosis and treatment seek to address the observed lesion, the quantified measurement, more than a person living in pain. The patient's own experience and subjective voice become inessential to the medical encounter. The experience many patients have of being ignored as a person, treated like a "thing," is not then just a matter of isolated insensitivity. It is symptomatic of a metaphysical position that has oriented modern medicine from the start. Just as medicine is beginning to acknowledge deficiencies in its atomistic understanding of illness and treatment, so too in its silencing of the patient's voice. When the patient is not treated as a living, desiring, suffering being, compliance is reduced, evidence is overlooked, inappropriate treatments are prescribed, genuine healing gives way to "fixing the machine."[81]

This presence of the corpse at the heart of Western medicine exposes the paradox in Descartes's strategy. For Descartes, death becomes the very tool that safeguards life, the means whereby disease is comprehended and mastered. The terror of the body inaugurated by the approach of first-person death is countered by the figure of the third-person corpse. For this body yields up all its secrets to the scientist/physician. Moreover, the shift from the first- to the third-person perspective makes death a less threatening thing. Bodily death becomes not my death exactly, but modeled first and foremost on that of the Other.[82] The true self cannot be threatened by the demise of that which from the start was mere mechanism. The dangerous body has been desubjectified, devitalized, demystified, by Cartesian science. The corporeal threat is, as far as possible, subdued.

6

To Form One Body

The great man regards Heaven and Earth and the myriad things as one body.
Wang Yang-ming, *Inquiry on the Great Learning*

The Phenomenological Vector

In these last two chapters I have suggested some of the experiential bases
for Cartesian dualism. Certain ontological presumptions are encouraged by the body's styles of absence: for example, the existence of the
reasoning mind as a separate, immaterial order of being. At the same
time, certain valuational schemas are suggested. The body, surfacing in
dys-appearance, comes to be associated with deception and death and is
consequently disvalued. The self is seen as fractured by an onto-valuational opposition.

I have suggested that the reasoning mind and the body are not in fact
opposing substances but intertwined aspects of one living organism.
Cartesian categories of mind and body merely reify and segregate classes of experience that stand in ceaseless interchange. Times in which the
body is most tacit and self-transcending are collected under the rubric
of rational "mind." Other experiences, where corporeality comes to
strong thematic presence, are collected under the rubric of "body." Yet,
as humans we are mentalized embodiment, now with an accent on transcendence or immanence, on self-forgetfulness or self-consciousness, on
projectivity or limitation.

This phenomenology, while undercutting the Cartesian reading,
also provides a way to account for it. It is true that splitting the self into
res cogitans and *res extensa* is incongruent with many aspects of lived
experience. As such, the Cartesian account is often assumed to arise
from metaphysical or epistemological commitments to the detriment of
attending to the life-world. I have suggested a different interpretation; it
is from the very immediacy of the life-world that this dualism is first
brought forth and by which it is continually sanctioned. The onto-valuational opposition of rational mind and body may be a misreading, but
one motivated by the lived body itself.

This is not meant to say that such a reading is mandated. Cartesianism, while resonating with doctrines held at other times and places,

is also a product of its specific sociohistorical context. We are acquainted with philosophies and cultures that assert the body as a positive force or as integrally imbued with mind. Such alternative interpretations draw upon their own domains of experiential support. The seeming immateriality of certain sorts of "minding" is offset by other modes wherein intelligence clearly resides right in the body. The educated hands of the musician or doctor constitute a striking example. Nor does the body surface only at dysfunctional moments. We have an ongoing, if subliminal, corporeal schema and kinesthetic sense that orients all our relations with the world. The body is a place not just of pain and illness but of cultivated pleasures, admired skills, health, sport, ornamentation, and ritual. The indefinite multiplicity of the body's employment allows for a wide variation in cultural interpretations of body.

Cartesian-style dualism is thus never an invariant, phenomenologically compelled by the structure of the lived body. However, the structure of embodiment does give rise to experiences that lend such a doctrine seeming support. Cartesian dualism thus rests upon what I will term a *phenomenological vector.*

What do I mean by this notion? It can best be explained with reference to Husserlian theory. For Husserl, the goal of phenomenology was to uncover the essences underlying the constitution of experience.[1] Through a process of variation, the investigator ascertains what remains constant and necessary throughout the range of an experiential field. While eschewing certain idealist strains in Husserl, my own work has been influenced by his methods; I have sought out existential/biological invariants that shape human experience. The ecstatic and recessive nature of the lived body is, I would suggest, one such invariant. That our senses operate with a "from-to" logic, that beneath the egoic "I" lies an anonymous visceral domain—such remains throughout the range of personal and cultural variations.

However, in addition to uncovering invariants, phenomenology can reveal what I will call vectors of meaning and use. A phenomenological vector is a structure of experience that makes possible and encourages the subject in certain practical or interpretive directions, while never mandating them as invariants.

I will illustrate this concept first by reference to the practical vectors established by the body's structure. Our fundamental anatomy and physiology delimit and suggest the modes of usage to which different corporeal regions will be put. For example, the hand is centrally employed in the labor of most cultures because of its high degree of plasticity, its freedom of action thanks to the upright posture and the dexterity of the opposable thumb. We also tend to use the hands when tactually exploring the world. The copious sensory innervation of this region allows for extraordinary tactile specificity. However, while such patterns of usage are encouraged by corporeal structure, they are neither necessary nor invariant. It is possible to imagine a culture that, given certain environmental or social conditions, would refocus many activities around the feet.

Similarly, the use of the mouth as an agent of primary communication is vectorial, not invariant. By virtue of its physiological capabilities, the mouth is peculiarly suited to the production of language. However, in sign language it is substituted for by the hands. For the most part, bodily praxis is articulated not according to essences but to vectors; our organs establish overlapping regions of possibilities, tendencies, and implied uses.

Moreover, such practical vectors are inevitably associated with vectors of interpretation. The body's structure and modes of employment suggest certain ways of interpreting body functions. For example, pain is often understood through models of sin, punishment, and evil. This clearly arises from the sensory aversiveness of pain. Though other hermeneutic possibilities remain, pain's unpleasant nature establishes a vector toward the negative. Another example, earlier mentioned, is the Western association of knowledge and vision. The ability of the eye to grasp and delineate vast regions of the world in simultaneous array suggests its gnostic preeminence within the panoply of the senses.

In this work, I have been arguing that Cartesian dualism itself trades upon interpretive vectors arising from the lived body. The sense of the understanding as immaterial is suggested by the disappearance from awareness of the brain, the signifier, the body of the thinker. Conversely, the sense of body as external threat is encouraged by the phenomenon of dys-appearance.

A phenomenological vector, in my usage, involves an ambiguous set of possibilities and tendencies that take on definite shape only within a cultural context. For example, the experience of dys-appearance may suggest the possibility of reading the body in a certain light, but it is in the discourses of a Plato, Augustine, or Descartes that this possibility is taken up and given precise discursive form. Ultimately, the very notion of a pure phenomenological vector somehow independent of its cultural manifestations is but an abstraction. The body's practices and self-interpretations are always already shaped by culture.

Conversely, culture is always shaped out of the stuff of bodies, arising in response to corporeal needs and desires. Food and housing must be secured, sexuality regulated, security ensured, dance and ritual organized. Body-based vectors are operative in shaping even the highest intellectual achievements of a culture. For example, Descartes's project of achieving a transcendent rationality is first suggested by the inherent finitude of embodied life. Only because our perceptions are necessarily limited, our lives involved with pain, illness, and death, does the Cartesian project have a telos.

Thus the vectors established by the lived body, and the cultural context in which they unfold, are mutually engendering structures. The human body shapes social practices, and social practices shape our use and understanding of the body. This can lead to what in engineering circles is termed a positive feedback loop. This is a situation where the outcome of a process is fed back into a system not to moderate but to augment its original direction of operation. It is as if a thermostat stimulated a boiler to stronger operation whenever it sensed the temperature was high. The room would soon be quite hot. I will claim that the interactive loop of body and culture has similarly "heated up" and intensified the Western predilection for dualism. A dualist metaphysics, first suggested by aspects of body experience, in turn feeds back to alter that experience, shifting it further in dualist directions.

I will illustrate this point first in relation to the notion of the immaterial intellect. Modes of corporeal disappearance, such as the hiddenness of the brain, the transparency of the sign, may suggest a model of disembodied rationality. However, once this model is accepted, usage and experience are further transformed in a "disembodied" direction. Not only are countervailing examples of embodied intelligence ignored, but they are systematically underdeveloped. The dominance of one corporeal vector can thus involve the repression of others.

The Western valorization of immaterial reason, dating back to the ancient Greeks, has shaped a variety of social practices. For example, Ihde contrasts Western sea navigation with that employed by the Polynesians,[2] who make use of perceptual information concerning cloud and light, wave patterns in the water, star movement, and the behavior of birds. This highly accurate navigational system clearly involves an embodied form of intelligence, encouraged by and encouraging an animistic view of world. By way of contrast, Western navigation is highly intellectualist, relying upon mathematical instruments and calculations. Such practices seem to support the belief that the book of nature is written in a geometrical language and available only to purified reason. (The Polynesians would be surprised.) A positive feedback loop is thus established. Our cultural belief in the disassociation of mind from body leads to an increase in disassociative practices; we are encouraged to abandon sensorimotor awareness for abstracted mathematical or linguistic forms. This in turn intensifies the day-to-day experience of mind as disembodied, confirming the initial cultural premise. As I sit here pursuing our socially sanctioned model of advanced intelligence—typing words on a computer screen—mind does seem like something disembodied indeed.

This positive feedback loop is even more evident relative to dys-appearance and the concept of body. The surfacing of the body at times of disruption may support a vector of threatening associations. However, once these are solidified into a negative discourse, there is a failure to pursue countervailing forms of positive body awareness. As discussed in chapter 4, such positive modes are largely optional in nature, dependent upon active seeking and cultivation. The Zen practice of meditation on the breath, the Tantric use of sexuality, the Yogic employment of physical postures, the development of martial arts and dance forms are but a few examples of the systematic enhancement of body experience more characteristic of Eastern cultures. Within such practices the body is viewed as a crucial medium of self-development and actualizes a variety of positive states of relaxation, concentration, coordination, ecstasy. Equivalent practices are by no means totally lacking in the West. However, those Western religious and philosophical traditions which adopt a largely negative view toward the body have placed a lesser emphasis upon cultivating its powers. The effect is to further skew our sense of body toward the negative. For, as has been seen, experiences of dys-appearance differ from other kinds of body awareness by virtue of their relatively compulsory nature. Whether attention is systematically developed or not, we have no choice but to remember the body when it screams out in pain, disrupts our projects with fatigue or lust, is wracked by disease, or threatened by death. If positive practices are shunned, such dysfunctional episodes can become the primary mode of body awareness, serving to define corporeality as a whole. Once again, this is the result of a positive feedback loop. A mistrust of the body engenders a neglect of salutary experiences, thereby skewing corporeal awareness further toward the negative and strengthening the original sense of body-as-threat.

Nor is this only a matter of insensitivity to the positive. This process can stimulate practices that forcibly intensify the negativity of body. For example, religious methods aimed at "subduing the flesh" by fierce asceticism may serve precisely to heighten the body's rebelliousness. Denied an outlet for its desires, the body surfaces as ever more demanding, ever more engaged in a battle against the will. A cultural assumption concerning the disobedience of body leads to subduing practices that serve to intensify and confirm its disobedience.[3] Nor is this point confined to ascetic practices. In more subtle ways, our ongoing cultural devaluation of the corporeal leads many of us to subject our bodies to excesses, abuses, and neglect that eventuate in illness and premature decline.

To use a Wittgensteinian metaphor, we have become trapped inside a picture.[4] A certain dualist picture has limited our self-development and self-relation. Moreover, this picture of onto-valuational dualism has deeply influenced our relations with others, emphasizing hierarchical opposition. For example, in our cultural hermeneutics, women have consistently been associated with the bodily sphere. They have been linked with nature, sexuality, and the passions, whereas men have been identified with the rational mind. This equation implicitly legitimizes structures of domination. Just as the mind is superior to and should rule the body, so men, it is suggested, should rule over women.[5]

The same terms can serve to justify class and labor inequities.[6] Lower-class workers are seen as just bodies who must be supervised by management "minds." An extreme and unequal division of labor is defended as natural through the metaphorics of dualism.

Our relation to other cultures has been shaped by much the same logic. Societies more obviously tied to the body and the earth are labeled as primitive and viewed with suspicion. The superior nature of Western rationality, with its literate, mathematical, and scientific modes, is all but assumed. The wisdom of tribal cultures is not recognized as such, or certainly not seen as of equal value.

This arrogance infects as well our relation to other species. If the mind or soul is identified primarily with intellection, then obviously animals do not have one. "Mindless" creatures can thus be viewed as inferior, or more extremely, as lacking any inherent worth. This ideology has been employed to justify all manner of appropriation, cruelty, and destruction directed toward nonhumans. Descartes's philosophy was thus used by the vivisectionists of his day to show that animals were incapable of suffering.[7]

Indeed, our relationship with nature as a whole has been reshaped by Cartesianism. Insofar as the earth was regarded as a living being, there were normative constraints on activities such as mining, which were seen as violations of her body.[8] But within Cartesianism the material world is a nonliving thing, devoid of intrinsic soul or telos. We are thus given unlimited license to reshape matter according to human desires. This can and does include strip mining, deforestation, indiscriminate development, and environmental pollution of all forms. The Cartesian conceptual "death of nature" thus helps lead to the real destruction of our ecosystem.

In all such cases, the hierarchical structure of onto-valuational dualism is used to validate modes of oppression. Certain individuals or groups are associated with the body. This includes women, laborers, "primitive" cultures, animals, and nature in general. They are thus defined as Other to the essential self, just as the body is Other. Moreover, insofar as the body is seen as mindless and in need of control, so too its representatives. Subjugation becomes a necessity and a natural prerogative.

Breaking free of this dualist picture is therefore a matter of no little cultural significance. But how do we do so? One method consists in simply criticizing the picture on logical and phenomenological grounds. There has been no lack of such efforts emanating from a variety of disciplines and perspectives. However, there can be a curious ineffectiveness to this direct approach. A picture may still continue to exert a powerful influence even after we have come to recognize its flaws. We must also recognize its strengths: that is, the ways in which it resonates with and illuminates aspects of human experience. We cannot escape from a picture until we understand the mechanisms whereby it has maintained its hold.

This is what I have attempted to accomplish in relation to Cartesian dualism. I have focused not on direct criticism of this model but on exposing certain of its experiential underpinnings. In this manner it is seen to deconstruct itself from within. Such tenets as the "disembodiment" of rationality are shown to arise precisely from the lived body. It is inherent in the structure of embodiment to self-conceal, to motivate misreadings. But when seen within the context of its origination, each misreading yields its kernel of truth. No longer a rallying cry for metaphysical hegemony, Cartesian notions of mind and body can be relativized into forms of description, articulating aspects of lived experience. Phenomenology becomes not just a tool for the refutation of previous philosophical positions but for their reinterpretation and reclamation.

At the same time phenomenology can also provide us with genuinely new ways of looking at the world. After all, we will rarely give up one picture unless we are offered a relevant and seemingly better alternative. The notion of the lived body, I believe, is such an alternative. It can help us to be more attentive to experience, uncover phenomena that were concealed, explain what the Cartesian framework renders inexplicable. However, a crucial question remains to be asked. I have suggested that one of the dangers of this dualist worldview is its tendency to give rise to hierarchical and oppressive social structures. But can the notion of the lived body here reorient our thinking? That is, can it serve as a framework for new values? Just as Cartesian dualism is an onto-valuational system, so the notion of the lived body can give rise to important social and ethical implications. I will close by addressing this matter.

I will not seek to treat this topic in a comprehensive form. Such would be another book on its own or a series of books. I intend merely to sketch out a potential line of thought, one that will doubtless raise as many questions as it answers. My goal is to provoke further discussion, not to foreclose it with conclusive argument.

In seeking inspiration on this subject it is helpful to step entirely outside of the Western tradition, dominated as it has been by onto-valuational dualisms. I will thus utilize a concept taken from Neo-Confucianism: namely, that we "form one body [t'i] with the universe." As ontology, the concept of "forming one body with the universe" echoes certain themes I have arrived at phenomenologically. As such, it will supply a nondualistic language with which to summarize my findings. Moreover, this Neo-Confucian concept is embedded within a rich discourse of values. "To form one body" is not simply an ontological statement but a moral/spiritual ideal meant to guide self-development. In seeking a new ethic, one appropriate to a recognition of the lived body, it will thus prove a suggestive source.

To Form One Body

Neo-Confucianism was a philosophical movement in China lasting roughly from the eleventh to the seventeenth centuries and synthesizing elements of Confucianism, Buddhism, and Taoism. A central theme is repeated in the work of several authors: namely, that there is an embodied unity of all things and, more particularly, of all things with the enlightened self. Thus Chang Tsai (1020–77) begins his influential "Western Inscription":

> Heaven is my father and Earth is my mother, and even such a small being as I finds an intimate place in their midst.
>   Therefore that which fills the universe I regard as my body and that which directs the universe I regard as my nature.[9]

Similarly, Ch'eng Hao (1032–85) comments:

> The man of *jen* [humanity] regards Heaven and Earth and all things as one body. To him there is nothing that is not himself.[10]

In Wang Yang-ming (1472–1529), one of the most important of the Neo-Confucian philosophers, this notion found its fullest expression. The *Inquiry on the Great Learning,* his central work, begins with the following discussion:

The great man regards Heaven and Earth and the myriad things as one body. He regards the world as one family and the country as one person . . . . That the great man can regard Heaven, Earth, and the myriad things as one body is not because he deliberately wants to do so, but because it is natural to the humane nature of his mind that he do so. Forming one body with Heaven, Earth, and the myriad things is not only true of the great man. Even the mind of the small man is no different.[11]

What is meant by this notion that all things form one body, and we with them? Like Cartesian dualism, it is an onto-valuational concept, speaking both of what is and of how things should be.

On the ontological plane, to say that all things "form one body" is to assert something about the fundamental structure of the universe as well as the place within it of human beings. According to the Neo-Confucian point of view, we are all composed of the same fundamental "stuff," or *ch'i*. *Ch'i* does not easily fit into Western dualistic categories. Neither solely spiritual nor material, *ch'i* has been translated variously as "vital force," "material force," "ether," or even "matter-energy." Historically, *ch'i* was regarded as a psychophysical power associated particularly with the blood and breath. Yet this same vital force is the substrate out of which all things arise from the most mundane to the most heavenly. As Tu Wei-ming, a twentieth-century commentator, writes:

Forming one body with the universe can literally mean that since all modalities of being are made of *ch'i,* human life is part of a continuous flow of the blood and breath that constitutes the cosmic process.[12]

We find ourselves in continuity with all things. Furthermore, this continuity sustains our life and well-being. Thus Wang Yang-ming writes:

Wind, rain, dew, thunder, sun and moon, stars, animals and plants, mountains and rivers, earth and stones are essentially of one body with man. It is for this reason that such things as the grains and animals can nourish man and that such things as medicine and minerals can heal diseases. Since they share the same material force [*ch'i*], they enter into one another.[13]

This concept of *ch'i* recalls in certain ways my treatment of the recessive dimension of the body. Supplementing Merleau-Ponty's discussion of the perceiving/perceived flesh, I referred to the "blood"—that visceral level whereby we are in chiasmatic relation to the organic world. One's body first arises from that of another, is composed of the same stuff as the surrounding world, and lives only by ceaseless metabolic exchanges with it. As such, we form one body with the universe we inhabit.

Just as the Neo-Confucian analysis acknowledges the recessive dimension of body, so too, its ecstasis. For Wang Yang-ming, we form one body with all things not simply because we share the same *ch'i:* we also do so by way of an expansive awareness through which we incorporate the surrounding world. The world is always given to us through our *hsin.* This Chinese notion, while usually translated as "mind," is not framed in opposition to corporeality. In Tu Wei-ming's words, *hsin* is "the most refined and subtle *ch'i* of the human body."[14] *Hsin* literally refers to the heart organ and is understood not only as the seat of consciousness and cognition but of affective and valuational response to the world.[15] Through this heart-mind awareness, especially when properly developed, we can experience and hence embody all things. As Hwa Yol Jung points out, Wang Yang-ming describes a correlativity of world and subject that anticipates the insights of existential phenomenology.[16] The world is an experienced world, its character dependent upon our powers of apprehension. Wang Yang-ming writes:

> If heaven is deprived of my clear intelligence, who is going to look into its height? If earth is deprived of my clear intelligence, who is going to look into its depth? . . . Separated from my clear intelligence, there will be no heaven, earth, spiritual beings, or myriad things, and separated from these, there will not be my clear intelligence.[17]

As the world exists only in relation to the experiencer, so the experiencer exists only in relation to the world.

> The eye has no substance of its own. Its substance consists of the colors of all things. The ear has no substance of its own. Its substance consists of the sound of all things. . . . The mind has no substance of its own. Its substance consists of the right or wrong of the influences and responses of Heaven, Earth, and all things.[18]

As subject, I do not inhabit a private theater of consciousness but am ecstatically intertwined, one body with the world.

There are thus convergences between Neo-Confucian ontology and the phenomenological account presented here. I form one body with the world because I am an ecstatic and recessive being.

It would be of interest to trace out in depth the similarities of and differences between these two conceptual systems. However, this is not my main intent. I wish to focus instead on the suggestiveness of this comparison vis-à-vis the domain of values. For Neo-Confucian ontology is always embedded within a matrix of moral/spiritual concerns.

The central question of these philosophers is never simply: What is the universe like? It is also: Given the nature of the universe, how can a human being become a "sage"—a fully realized person?

That these two questions are so closely associated suggests that the fact-value distinction, central to contemporary Western thought, is foreign to the Neo-Confucian mind. Moral ideals are seen to flow directly out of the structure of the cosmos. Insofar as it is an ontological truth that we "form one body" with the universe, it is a moral imperative that we live in accordance with this principle. However, the Neo-Confucian recognizes that we often fail to do so. Only the sage truly *realizes* this structure of communion, that is, makes it experientially real by embodying it in day-to-day concerns. For most of us, our separative ego and selfish desires seem far more real than any universal bonds. When one thus lives for oneself in denial of relation, there is no limit to the conflict and brutality that can result. As Wang Yang-ming writes, such a man:

> will destroy things, kill members of his own species, and will do everything. In extreme cases he will even slaughter his own brothers, and the humanity that forms one body will disappear completely.[19]

How then do we realize in our daily lives the truth of universal interconnectedness? For Wang Yang-ming, it is *not* a matter of overcoming natural selfishness through a process of social training. Rather, interconnectedness is innate to the heart-mind. This is evidenced by the human propensity for compassionate identification. Such is a part of everyone's nature, sage or not.

> Even the mind of the small man is no different. . . . Therefore when he sees a child about to fall into a well, he cannot help a feeling of alarm and commiseration. This shows that his humanity forms one body with the child. It may be objected that the child belongs to the same species. Again, when he observes the pitiful cries and frightened appearance of birds and animals about to be slaughtered, he cannot help feeling an "inability to bear" their suffering. This shows that his humanity forms one body with birds and animals. It may be objected that birds and animals are sentient beings as he is. But when he sees plants broken and destroyed, he cannot help a feeling of pity. This shows that his humanity forms one body with plants. It may be said that plants are living things as he is. Yet, even when he sees tiles and stones shattered and crushed, he cannot help a feeling of regret. This shows that his humanity forms one body with tiles and stones. This means that even the mind of the small man necessarily has the humanity that forms one body with all.[20]

Our consanguineous relation with all things finds expression in intuitive empathy. Selfish desires are pernicious because they have the power to obscure, like clouds the sun, our innate and immediate compassion.[21] Thus the training of the sage consists entirely in the clearing away of selfish desire, not the inculcation of anything new.[22] This allows one's innate knowledge and compassion to reemerge. Through a loving identification with and nurturance of all things, the sage then forms one body with the universe. An ontological principle is existentially realized.

Such a vision may seem remote from the debates of contemporary ethics. But I would suggest that it lays the groundwork for a new ethic of embodiment. Insofar as the Cartesian notion of body is rooted in phenomena of dys-appearance, an ethic of transcending or controlling the body is a natural consequence. If the body is associated primarily with dysfunction and limitation, then the victorious life demands its overcoming. This fundamental project played itself out and continues today in the spheres of epistemology, politics, morals, and medicine.

However, as has been noted above, dys-appearance is a derivative phenomenon. The body stands out at times of dysfunction only because its usual state is to be lost in the world—caught up in a web of organic and intentional involvements through which we form one body with other things. To say that the body is "absent," a "being-away," thus has a positive significance; it asserts that the body is in ceaseless relation to the world. As recessive being, these worldly relations are organic and preconscious. As ecstatic being, we are in conscious and purposive intercourse with the environment. There is a two-sided linkage, flesh and blood, ecstatic and recessive, each dimension of engagement mirroring the other. I gaze up at the stars . . . at the same time I know that the carbon molecules from which my body is made were forged in the furnace of dying stars. I am thus doubly connected to even the far reaches of the universe. We form one organic/perceptual circuit.[23]

If the Cartesian vision of body-as-threat encouraged an ethic of corporeal repression, then this new vision of the body can encourage a cultivation of embodied relation. As with the Neo-Confucians, we are invited to realize those possibilities of communion which lie implicit in the prethematic structure of the body.[24] This is not to claim that such an ethic is required by my findings or the evidence of experience. To use my previous term, the notion of forming one body is an interpretive vector; it is a way of understanding embodied life made possible and fostered by phenomenological structures. The profound interconnection between body and world invites an ontology and ethics of interconnection. But an interpretive vector is only suggested by experience, never compelled. The body can always be viewed in a multiplicity of ways, with a focus on separation or connection, finitude or transcendence, stability or change.

This is not to say, however, there are not better or worse interpretive structures. Does an ontology and ethics exhibit the revelatory power to disclose what was concealed? Can it integrate diverse phenomena and bring aesthetic coherence to our vision of world? Does it supply a vision of the good life that can inspire personal and social change? Does it speak to the problems facing the culture? Can it provide a corrective to the practical and conceptual failures of previous systems? On all such scores I think the Neo-Confucian model is a worthy successor to Cartesianism.[25]

But what would it mean concretely to cultivate the principle of forming one body? In exploring this question I will begin with but go beyond the Neo-Confucian interpretation. I will suggest that this principle can be realized through a variety of modalities, somewhat different in their emphasis, though closely intertwined. In the explicitly moral sphere, we can speak, like Wang Yang-ming, of forming one body through *compassion* for others. Yet we may also form one body through aesthetic openness to the world. I will refer to this as the experience of *absorption.* Then too, there are spiritual practices designed to facilitate interconnection with the ground of all being. These yield what I will term the experience of *communion.* Compassion, absorption, communion—in each case, we realize the one-body relation. My distinction between these moral, aesthetic, and spiritual modes is meant only as provisional, not absolute. These are modulations on a common theme, expressions of a unifying principle.

Compassion

The moral significance of forming one body is clearly revealed by the experience of compassion. As already seen, the Neo-Confucians found in compassion the existential bond whereby the individual realized his/her communion with the whole. The word compassion is derived from the Latin *cum* and *patior,* which together can be literally translated as "to suffer with." Indeed, we ordinarily speak of extending compassion to one who is undergoing suffering of some sort. However, the Latin notion of *patior* is not used solely in reference to pain and misfortune; more broadly, it means to suffer something to happen, that is, to undergo an experience.[26] I use *compassion* in this sense as a general term that refers to an experiencing-with, whether it takes the form of sharing another's sorrow or joy, mourning together, or partaking in communal celebration.[27] In each case we enter into the experience of others through a process of empathic identification.

The experience of compassion is never reducible to a set of judgments and behavioral dispositions. For example, when visiting a friend in her sickbed, I may have a cognitive awareness that she is suffering and decide to place myself at her disposal. I try to distract her from her pain with cheerful conversation and offer to bring her food, drink, or fresh pillows. Having understood that she is in discomfort, I have taken the appropriate beneficent measures. And yet compassion may be wholly lacking. For in this situation I can do and say "the right thing" without ever embodying the Other's experience. Her face, contorted and tearful, remains a surface in the world, not that which reveals to me a depth of experience. Her suffering does not awaken a mutual resonance in my being. I am cold, preoccupied with my private concerns, even as she is preoccupied with hers. I have not "put myself in her place," incorporated her perspective. We form two bodies.

Yet one can imagine an existential shift. Perhaps, in the midst of my hollow pleasantries, my friend lets out an involuntary moan. Suddenly my words fall away and something opens up within me. I look into her eyes and, as if for the first time, truly *see* her suffering. The other person comes alive to me; she becomes real, dimensional, a living, breathing person just as I am. I begin to feel something of her suffering, her fear and frustration. These awaken an echo of the same within me. My eyes moisten as we speak. In a sense, these are her tears now inhabiting my body for I have begun to see the world as if through her eyes. Compassion has made one body of us.

This does not imply that all distinction between us is eradicated. As Scheler points out, to experience true sympathy for others (*Mitgefuhl*), it is necessary to retain a sense of their otherness.[28] I feel *for* my friend; if I am completely taken over by her experience such that our identities blur, I can no longer speak of concernful relation. Moreover, our bodily structure itself prohibits total identification. To be embodied is to inhabit a particular place and time, to have a unique history, physiology, and perceptual perspective. Our bodies mark us off as unmistakably different even as they open us up to interconnection. I am not my sick friend lying in her hospital bed, though I have incorporated a portion of her suffering.

To speak of forming one body is thus never meant to deny difference but, rather, to assert the truth of relation. Through compassion we actualize a "oneness" in the sense of Merleau-Pontian chiasm, a coiling circuit of connection between divergent terms. Just as I am in perceptual chiasm with my friend, so there is a "chiasm of the heart" that joins us affectively. To become aware of and deepen this concernful linkage is to realize ontological relatedness; my friend and I belong to one flesh and blood.

The embodied root of this compassionate bond is suggested in a variety of languages. The Hebrew term for compassion, *rachamim,* is derived from the word for womb or bowels. In the Jewish Bible, God's own bowels are said to be troubled by concern for others (e.g., Jeremiah 31:20).[29] We find a similar sense in the New Testament use of the Greek verb *splangchnizomai,* "to be moved with compassion." The *splangchna* are the viscera, such as heart and entrails, regarded as the center of our most intense emotions. This term is applied only to Jesus and his Father throughout the New Testament Gospels.[30] The sacred ideal in such texts is not one in which the body is overcome but in which it reverberates lovingly with those of others. There is a "gut level" identification with the feelings of those around us.

Compassion actualizes the one-body state not only through this affective bond but by the actions that follow. The natural expression of compassion is service. Insofar as I embody within myself the suffering and needs of others, it follows naturally that I will seek to alleviate these sufferings and fulfill these needs. They are, in an important sense, mine. Swami Ramdas describes this from the Hindu perspective:

> Just as a flower gives out its radiance to whomsoever approaches or uses it, so love from within us radiates toward everybody and manifests as spontaneous service. . . . When we feed, clothe and attend on anybody, we feel like doing all these things to our own body, for which we do not expect any return or praise or commendation, because all bodies are our own; for, we as the all-pervading Atman or Spirit reside in all bodies.[31]

Thus, one-body compassion for my sick friend leads me to do what I can for her: hold her hand, offer words of comfort, bring her food, fix her bedclothes. I give over my motoric possibilities to be guided by her desires. If she is thirsty, my hands fetch her drink. If she is weak, my limbs supply her strength. We act as if we were one functioning body, her "I can" supplemented by my abilities, her wishes fulfilled by my work. It is this embracing of relation as much as the specific actions I perform, that brings about the relief of suffering. For her suffering is based partially in the experience of isolation. As I discussed, pain and disease disrupt communion with the natural and social world, creating a lived solipsism. When another consents to form one body even with the ill body—one in pain, contorted, or disabled—this exerts a healing force. The isolation imposed by illness is somewhat overcome.

Though I have begun by discussing a relation between two people, this empathic bond can be indefinitely extended. I may seek to serve the needs of my family, my community, my country, all human beings, the world at large. Compassionate connection thus expands outward in concentric circles of identification. In each case I form an ever larger body through joining my welfare, desires, and abilities with those of others.

We thus speak of governing bodies, the mystical body of the church, the body politic, *corpor*ations, and the like.

The ideal to which the Neo-Confucians point, as do many spiritual traditions, is that state in which we form one body with *all things*. To explain how we may achieve universal empathy despite the particularity of human ties, Wang Yang-ming uses the image of a branching tree.[32] A tree must have a solid root to grow. In this case, the root is that love we feel for those to whom we are closest, as love between father and son, or elder and younger brother. But as the root gives rise to a trunk, and that to branches and leaves, so our compassion can gradually extend to all.

> Everything from ruler, minister, husband, wife, and friends to mountains, rivers, spiritual beings, birds, animals, and plants should be truly loved in order to realize my humanity that forms one body with them, and then my clear character will be completely manifested, and I will really form one body with Heaven, Earth, and the myriad things.[33]

This extension of compassion even to the nonhuman world is somewhat foreign to the Judeo-Christian tradition.[34] There, "love of neighbor" has usually been interpreted as referring exclusively to human neighbors. More embracing visions have surfaced from time to time. Thus, St. Francis lovingly addresses Brother Sun and Sister Moon, Brother Wind and Sister Water, Brother Fire and Mother Earth.[35] All nature, in this image, is consanguineous. Martin Buber similarly suggests that we can realize the I-Thou moment even in our relations to the nonhuman sphere.[36] Yet this sense of compassionate mutuality with nature is the exception rather than the rule in the West. This in turn has had practical ramifications, as evidenced by our ravaged environment and ecological crises.[37] There seems a pressing need for a more embracing moral ideal, one that extends beyond an interhuman concern. Admittedly, our forms of identification and moral commitment will vary in relation to different entities. But to exclude nature entirely from the moral sphere—to consider it in the Cartesian mode as mere *res extensa*—is to risk vitiating or destroying our world. The Neo-Confucian model has no such exclusions. We are challenged to form one body with all things.

Absorption

The one-body principle finds expression not only in moral but aesthetic experience. A compassionate concern for others is one way of opening to the world. But we also open through an aesthetic sensitivity to things, be it a landscape, a work of art, or the objects of our everyday life. Ordinarily, many of us are relatively oblivious to our surroundings. Yet there are times when we awaken and the world rushes in, fraught with beauty or significance. At such times, we truly become *absorbed* in our world. That such absorption is a deeply embodied process is suggested by the word itself. It derives from the Latin root *sorbere* meaning to "suck in" or "swallow." When we become deeply absorbed, as in a natural landscape, it is as if we were swallowed into a larger body. At the same time, this landscape is swallowed into our embodiment, transforming it from within. There is a bidirectional incorporation. The following example may help illustrate this point.

I am walking down a forest path. Yet, I am not attending to my world in a bodily or mindful way. I am caught up in my own worries—a paper that needs completion, a financial problem. My thoughts are running their private race, unrelated to the landscape. I am dimly aware of the sights and sounds of nature, but it is a surface awareness. The landscape neither penetrates into me, nor I into it. We are two bodies.

Yet, once again, it is possible to imagine an existential shift. Over time, through the rhythm of my walking, the calmness of the scene, my mind begins to quiet. Something catches my ear—the trilling of a bird. I glance up in time to see the bird hopping from branch to branch, its bright colors shining in the sunlight. I gradually become aware of other birds, other songs, and, as if awakening from a dream, realize that I stand in the midst of a wild chorus. I am beginning to absorb the world around me and become absorbed in it. My expanded awareness now roams across the landscape: from the birds to the green beauty of the trees, the sunlight dappling the leaves, their windblown rustling, the sound of water in the distance, the warmth of the sun on my cheek.

This aesthetic absorption is a mode of one-body relation. I open feelingly such that the world can penetrate my senses, my muscles, my consciousness. The temporality of the landscape transforms my temporality. The slow crescendo and decrescendo of the wind, the stately glide of clouds awaken a resonance within my body-mind such that my hurried stride begins to slow, my thoughts to glide effortlessly, no longer rushing toward a goal. The spaciousness of the outdoors becomes my space. I somehow begin having bigger ideas than the cramped concerns that preoccupied me. From my broader perspective I can see the smallness of my previous worries. New thoughts form within me that I have never had in my windowless office. They feel *in-spired,* "breathed in" as if from the wind and trees. Then too, I may find my mind settling into unaccustomed silence. Where before there were words and more words, now there are only bird calls and the whispering of leaves.

The boundaries between inner and outer thus become porous. As I close my eyes I feel the sun and hear the bird songs both within-me-without-me. They are not sense data internal to consciousness, but neither are they "out there" somewhere. They are part of a rich body-world chiasm that eludes dualistic characterizations. My relaxation *is* the smell of pine needles and the warmth of the breeze; self and Other can only be artificially disentangled. It is by this bodily chiasm that I realize the height of a distant tree. Though I am planted here in my puny frame, I am there too at the peak, towering one hundred feet high. I am likewise with the bird's graceful flight, the brook tumbling over logs and stones. This is an experience of bidirectional incorporation; the world comes alive empathically within my body, even as I experience myself as part of the body of the world.

Such moments have an ecstatic quality, bringing a feeling of joyful release. As we have seen, the surface body is always an ecstatic structure, standing out from itself through its sensorimotor involvements. But such aesthetic experiences, like those of compassion, help us to realize this expansive being. In the ecstasy that comes upon us in the woods, we feel the leaping beyond constriction, the spaciousness of our extended body. We register our flesh-and-blood chiasm with the world.

This aesthetic incorporation is by no means restricted to experiences of nature. It is there when we enter deeply into a work of art. We may skim past a hundred canvases before we become *absorbed* in one. Its mood then starts to saturate our being, its sense of space and time, of rhythm and beauty. How we see the world is subtly shifted as we incorporate the artist's gaze. Nor is this aesthetic incorporation confined to the contemplative rather than the practical sphere. It is not merely the art appreciator who realizes ecstatic involvement but the artist as well, in her or his full-bodied engagement with landscape, canvas, and paint. And while the contemplative walker may embody the forest, so too, in a different way, may the one who works the wood. Heidegger thus writes of a cabinetmaker's apprentice:

> If he is to become a true cabinetmaker, he makes himself answer and respond above all to the different kinds of wood and to the shapes slumbering within wood—to wood as it enters into man's dwelling with all the hidden riches of its nature. In fact, this relatedness to wood is what maintains the whole craft.[38]

The cabinetmaker's hands must become sensitively absorbed in the body of the wood—its grain, texture, knots and curves—just as the wood comes to absorb the skill of these hands. There is a corporeal intertwining at the heart of such a craft.

I have dwelt so far on experiences involving the natural world, art, or crafted objects. I could extend this discussion to a variety of domains:

for example, there are modes of absorption actualized in sexuality, in sports, even in certain forms of doing science. Yet a question would still remain. The Neo-Confucian ideal that has guided our inquiry is that of forming one body *with all things*. But when we encounter this in the mode of aesthetic absorption it seems we are driven toward selectivity. Can we open to the one-body experience just as much in a parking lot as in the woods? Are there not certain environments that invite us to ecstatic participation and others that naturally foreclose this experience?

A twofold reply is in order. It has been suggested by the world's spiritual literature that the realized sage can, indeed, open appreciatively to all the world, including within it suffering, disruption, the ordinary, and the downright ugly. Each is found to have its place in the harmony of the all. The beauty of the commonplace, for example, is emphasized in Zen aesthetics. Tea drinking was elevated to a Zen art form not because of its exoticism but precisely because it is such an ordinary act. At its limit, we can imagine an aesthetic openness to any and all environments, just as we can imagine extending compassion to any and all beings.

Nonetheless, for most of us, the extent to which we can open feelingly to the world depends upon the world in which we find ourselves. The assault of concrete and jackhammers does not invite embodied involvement as does a forest glade. Assembly line work does not elicit the skillful sensitivity to materials that is intrinsic to fine crafts.[39] Because we *do* form one body with the world, like it or not, such dehumanized environments will have their impact on our nerves and hearts. But because this impact is experienced as unpleasant and intrusive, we are driven to avoid the one-body relation, not to realize it. That is, we seek to shut down cognitively, emotionally, perceptually, to alienated environments. Thus, to stimulate the realization of one-bodied relation, we need to cultivate a world that encourages our involvement. What such a world would be like is open to competing visions: some might emphasize the conservation of wilderness, others, the humanization of our cities; some, the eradication of ghetto poverty, others, the provision of challenging work. In each case, there is an attempt to maintain or construct an environment which invites mindful/bodily participation.

Communion

In my previous discussions of compassion and absorption I began with experiences of limited focus. One opens feelingly to a suffering friend or to the beauty of a natural landscape. I then pointed toward the ideal of forming one body *with all things*. As Wang Yang-ming suggests, the love for a parent can be the root of a tree that eventually bears fruit in the love for all. Similarly, a beautiful painting can be the instrument that awakens us to the beauty of the world. But such expansive vision, if it is to last more than a passing moment, is dependent upon systematic, almost heroic, development. For most of us, compassion and absorption remain confined to highly circumscribed regions. We feel love for a particular person and not another, truly attend to an artwork but not to the ordinary. We do not form one body with all things.

Yet there are practices expressly designed to facilitate a sense of involvement with the All, however that is defined and understood. These practices are to be found at the heart of the world's spiritual traditions and take the form of ritual, prayer, meditation, and the like. The experiences encouraged by such practices, though highly diverse, I will cluster under the term *communion*. To experience communion, in this usage, is to realize a relationship to that which is felt to be the ground of being, whether this be called God, Brahman, Suchness, the Tao, or any of an indefinite list of names. I choose the term *communion* both for its resonances with "union" or oneness, and its historic association with sacred practice.[40*]

Within the West, spiritual experience has often been thought of as divorced from, or opposed to, the bodily sphere. The Cartesian understanding of body-as-threat draws upon a long philosophical/theological tradition. If the body is identified with dysfunction and separation it must be transcended, repressed, or otherwise overcome for the self to realize relation with the All. This model has by now been widely criticized. It can lead to inordinate hatred of the body and its passions. It can also blind us to the import within the spiritual life of bodily practices and physical environments. These arguments have been presented at length by other authors.[41] I will not belabor the point here. Instead I will pursue the alternate account implicit in the notion of forming one body. The very phrase suggests that corporeality is not simply an obstacle to spiritual experience but can be central to its realization.

This is perhaps most clearly exemplified by religious ritual. As Zuesse writes:

> Ritual centers on the body, and if we would understand ritual we shall have to take the body seriously as a vehicle for religious experience. . . . Much ritual symbolism draws on the simplest and most intense sensory experiences, such as eating, sexuality, and pain. Such experiences have been repeated so often or so intimately by the body that they have become primary forms of bodily awareness. In ritual, they are transformed into symbolic experiences of the divine, and even into the form of the cosmic drama itself.[42]

I will take as an illustration the Christian ritual of the Eucharist. This unfolds through a bodily intertwining of priest or minister, bread and wine, Christ, and the community of celebrants.

In first consecrating the offerings, the priest or minister repeats Christ's language from the Last Supper. There is an intertwining as Christ's own words, spoken almost two thousand years ago, now flow through the body of another. Yet this sacred presence, as mediated by language, remains incomplete. The words are intangible, a disappearing body. The presence of Christ is given substance through the bread and wine. These are objects to be seen, handled, tasted. They further incarnate a flesh-and-blood presence, whether this presence is theologically interpreted as symbolic or real.

Moreover, the bread and wine enable one to enter into a visceral relation with the divine. Up until this point the sacred has been accessed through the sensorimotor body: the sight of vaulting arches leading the gaze up to heaven, the harmonies of sacred music, the humility engendered by bent knee and lowered head. But now the divine penetrates even one's inner body. As food and drink, the sacred merges with the worshipper, sustaining and nourishing from within. Through this incorporation one realizes an intimate intertwining with the divine. So too, is there an intertwining with the community of celebrants. All present have been nourished by the same bodily/spiritual meal. By extension, they eat side by side, in embodied relation, with all who belong to the Christian faith. As Paul writes, "Because there is one loaf, we who are many are one body, for we all partake of the one loaf" (1 Corinthians 10:17).

This ritual, like all rituals, can quickly become a hollow thing, a mere set of actions performed out of duty. However, for the attentive Christian, it can also become a vehicle for profound one-body experience. This experience may be modulated in different directions, depending on the individual and the form of eucharistic celebration. For some, the closeness with other celebrants is key. The shared meal is alive with resonances of family, festivity, and intimacy. This may be accentuated when there is an actual breaking of one bread and a drinking from one goblet. For others, the experience is of individual relation to Christ. No one else, after all, can do one's own eating and drinking. Prior to taking communion, one may sense Christ as somewhere else than where one sits: a being who resides up in Heaven or out there on the altar. But swallowing the host can inaugurate a shift. Now Christ dwells within. God is no longer a remote figure but someone incarnated inside one's own heart bringing a renewed sense of strength and joy. One may find oneself thinking more Christ-thoughts, feeling Christ-love lighting up one's soul. One leaves church in an expanded state. While incorporating the Eucharist, one has also been incorporated by it, opening to a wider source of love and awareness.

For many Christians this one-body relation is consonant with irreducible difference. Though Christ may be the living fire that sparks one's own soul, they would not view themselves, strictly speaking, as identical with him. Rather, the divine is understood as a being to whom one stands in relation, properly that of obedience and love. This may be referred to as the *devotional* form of communion. But also ingredient in the world's spiritual traditions is what might be termed the *mystical* communion.[43] Here the one-body experience takes a somewhat different form. It is not primarily a matter of devotion to, but of an identification with, the All. The distinction between the self and the Ultimate falls away in the face of profound unitive experiences.

As an example of a practice geared to actualize this mode, I will turn to Zen meditation. This practice is a far cry from what I have just been discussing. Whereas the meaning of the Eucharist depends on a complex theology, Zen eschews metaphysical explanation along with the notion of a personal God. And while the ritual of the Eucharist unfolds as a communal ceremony, Zen meditation involves a rigorous going within. Yet it is no less an example of one-body communion.

This can be seen both in the unitive awareness toward which Zen practice leads and the emphasis within this practice on correct embodiment. Unlike the Christian ritual, which infuses something pure into the body, Zen purifies the body/mind by a stripping away. In order to realize enlightenment, we must rid ourselves of those modes of acting and thinking which reinforce duality. According to Zen, we constantly divide reality into "this" versus "that," good versus bad, self versus Other. We are left clinging to the illusion of a personal "I," which must grasp at certain things and push other things away. This "I" will never be at home in its world. It is always threatened by pain and extinction.

In meditation, one begins to suspend, examine, and overcome this separative body/mind. Where perception ordinarily leads to desire, desire to action, and action to new perceptions and desires, the cycle is broken for the meditator. He or she simply sits. Attention is drawn away from outer-perception; the room should be quiet, the light not too bright, the eyes half-closed and unfocused. All movement is suspended. If an urge arises one notes it but does not pursue it. Even the annoying itch is left unscratched, the fly left free to buzz around the face. This allows one to unify and concentrate the lived body, not disperse it in outer action. To this end, one's legs are interlaced in the lotus position, one's hands brought together in the "cosmic mudra." The spine is kept straight, weight and breathing centered in the lower abdomen, all geared toward realizing a relaxed alertness.

In the Soto manner of Zen, attention is then turned to the act of breathing. Why this? For one, the rise and fall of the breath serves as a repetitive and calming stimulus. It also establishes a neutral focus that frees one up from customary thought structures; each time a worry or desire arises one simply brings attention back to the breath. However, these purposes could be accomplished by almost any constant or repetitive stimulus. There is something more about breathing that makes it a potent tool for surpassing dualism.

Physiologically, respiration stands at the very threshold of the ecstatic and visceral, the voluntary and involuntary. While we can modulate our breathing at will, it is primarily an automatic function. The meditator finds that he or she "is breathed" as much as the breather. Watching the breath come in and go out for minutes or hours, one is saturated by the presence of a natural power that outruns the "I." Breathing simply happens and happens and happens. There is no need for willful management; all is accomplished without effort on one's part. Thus, breathing becomes the very prototype of Zen/taoist *wu-wei*, literally translated as "non-action." This term refers to the effortless acting typical of one who has broken free from ego-identification. If meditation is regular and persistent, this consciousness may remain when one has arisen from the mat. One cleans the dishes, but it is as if breathing. One speaks with a friend, but it is as if breathing. All unfolds with a natural and effortless rhythm. Who after all is doing the breathing, cleaning, talking? Not "I."

There is yet another way in which meditation on the breath can carry one beyond the separative ego. Moment to moment, breathing actualizes our one-body relation with the surrounding world. Zen master Shunryu Suzuki addresses his students:

> When we practice zazen our mind always follows our breathing. When we inhale, the air comes into the inner world. When we exhale, the air goes out to the outer world. The inner world is limitless, and the outer world is also limitless. We say "inner world" or "outer world," but actually there is just one whole world. In this limitless world, our throat is like a swinging door. The air comes in and goes out like someone passing through a swinging door. If you think, "I breathe," the "I" is extra. There is no you to say "I." What we call "I" is just a swinging door which moves when we inhale and when we exhale.[44]

Inside and outside, self and Other, are relativized, porous, each time one takes a breath. The air is constantly transgressing boundaries, sustaining life through interconnection. One may have spent years studying the mystics on the unreality of dualism, and have this remain but an abstract idea. But in following the breath one begins to *embody* this truth.

The unitive consciousness built through this or other forms of meditation reaches shocking fulfillment in the moment of satori. As a Zen description goes, "I came to realize clearly that Mind is no other than mountains and rivers and the great wide earth, the sun and the moon and the stars."[45] In the mystical communion, self and world are realized as one. Accounts of the enlightenment experience give some sense of the joyful explosion involved. There is frequently laughter, spontaneity, a feeling of ecstatic release, an expansive sense of love and harmony. A Canadian housewife describes some of her experience thusly:

> When I am in solitude I can hear a "song" coming forth from everything. Each and everything has its own song; even moods, thoughts, and feelings have their finer songs. Yet beneath this variety they intermingle in one inexpressibly vast unity.
>
> I feel a love which, without object, is best called lovingness. But my old emotional reactions still coarsely interfere with the expressions of this supremely gentle and effortless lovingness.
>
> I feel a consciousness which is neither myself nor not myself, which is protecting or leading me into directions helpful to my proper growth and maturity, and propelling me away from that which is against that growth. It is like a stream into which I have flowed and, joyously, is carrying me beyond myself.[46]

Here can be seen the one-body experience modulated into its various keys. There is a sense of heightened aesthetic absorption in the "song" emanating from all things; of loving compassion without limit; of communion with a sacred ground of being. This communion involves a mystical core, the intuition of the "inexpressibly vast unity" of all. Yet there remains in this case a devotional element, seen in the reference to a consciousness not wholly herself.

In the ritual of the Eucharist, eating and drinking become a vehicle for incorporating the divine. In Zen, an embodiment of stillness and breath helps throw one beyond ego-identification. In each case the lived body can unlock realization of the transpersonal only because *it already is a transpersonal thing*. In eating, breathing, perceiving, moving, the body transcends itself through its commerce with the world. Thus, each visceral or sensorimotor function can become a channel for the experience of communion. Some practices use sound in such a way: chanting "Om" for example, the sound in which all sounds are said to be contained, or listening to the modulations of a Gregorian chant. Other practices focus on the eye. This is apparent in the Tibetan and Native

American use of mandalas or the heavenly spires of a medieval cathedral. In each instance, through perceiving a sensuous symbol we experience our relatedness to the All. Other practices make use of movement, as in the Sufi dance of the whirling dervishes. The ecstasis of motion is intensified until it transfigures into a means of self-transcendence. Similarly, the union realized in sexuality becomes a Tantric tool for surpassing duality. Almost all spiritual traditions use posture and gesture as a means whereby we enter into relation with the divine. The Christian kneels in humility, the Jew stands in respectful prayer, the Moslem prostrates in submission and adoration. We thus take embodied regard for that which is larger and greater than the self.

The Cartesian model cannot fully account for such practices. For therein the body is seen as a force of deception and limitation and ontologically identified with sheer *presence*. It is an object with clearly defined location and boundaries, here, not there, enclosed within itself. But I have focused throughout this work on the *absence* of the lived body, its being-away. This body's roots reach down into the soil of an organismic vitality where the conscious mind cannot follow. Its branches spread throughout the universe. When I gaze upon the stars, or the face of another, or the symbols of divinity, I transgress my limits. Through the lived body I open to the world. This body is not then simply a mass of matter or an obstructive force. It is a way in which we, as part of the universe, mirror the universe.

It is a jewel in Indra's net.

Notes

Notes marked with an asterisk (*) indicate places where I have taken up significant issues not treated within the main text.

Introduction

1. J. H. van den Berg, "The Human Body and the Significance of Human Movement," *Philosophy and Phenomenological Research* 13 (1952):169.

2. See, for example, Jacques Derrida, *Speech and Phenomena,* trans. David B. Allison (Evanston, Ill.: Northwestern University Press, 1973).

3. Robert Sokolowski, *Presence and Absence* (Bloomington: Indiana University Press, 1978).

4. Maurice Merleau-Ponty, *The Visible and the Invisible,* ed. Claude Lefort, trans. Alphonso Lingis (Evanston, Ill.: Northwestern University Press, 1968).

5. Maurice Merleau-Ponty, *Phenomenology of Perception,* trans. Colin Smith (London and Henley: Routledge and Kegan Paul, 1962), pp. 80–97.

6. Merleau-Ponty, *Phenomenology of Perception.*

7. Ibid., pp. 346–65, and Merleau-Ponty, *The Visible and the Invisible,* pp. 130–55.

8. See Patrick Heelan, *Space-perception and the Philosophy of Science* (Berkeley and Los Angeles: University of California Press, 1983).

9. Merleau-Ponty, *Phenomenology of Perception,* pp. 174–99, 383–92, and *The Visible and the Invisible,* pp. 149–55.

Chapter One: The Ecstatic Body

1. Maurice Merleau-Ponty, *The Structure of Behavior,* trans. Alden L. Fisher (Boston: Beacon Press, 1963), p. 213.

2. See Merleau-Ponty, *Phenomenology of Perception,* p. 90.

3. See Jean-Paul Sartre, *Being and Nothingness,* trans. Hazel E. Barnes (New York: Washington Square Press, 1966), pp. 418–19.

4. Merleau-Ponty, *The Structure of Behavior,* p. 217.

5. Ibid.

6. Merleau-Ponty, *Phenomenology of Perception,* p. 101.

7. Edmund Husserl, *Ideen zu einer reinen Phänomenologie und phänomenologischen Philosophie,* Book 2. *Phänomenologische Untersuchungen zur Konstitution,* ed. Marly Biemel, *Husserliana,* vol. 4 (The Hague: Martinus Nijhoff, 1952), p. 158.

8. See Donn Welton, "Soft Smooth Hands: Husserl's Phenomenology of the Lived-Body," State University of New York at Stony Brook, 1986. Typescript.

9. Sartre, *Being and Nothingness,* p. 402.

10. This is not to say that there is an ontological difference that divides the seeing eye from the eye-as-seen. While Sartre, with his dualistic predilections, does imply such an ontological division, the later Merleau-Ponty stresses the "reversibility" of the seeing and the seen as poles of a single ontological circuit of the "Visible" (see my chapter 2).

11. Merleau-Ponty, *Phenomenology of Perception,* p. 92.

12. Husserl, *Ideen 2,* p. 145.

13. Merleau-Ponty, *The Visible and the Invisible,* pp. 147–48. Also see Merleau-Ponty, *Phenomenology of Perception,* p. 92.

14. See Erwin Straus, *The Primary World of Senses,* trans. Jacob Needleman (Glencoe, N.Y.: The Free Press of Glencoe, 1963), pp. 367–79, and *Phenomenological Psychology,* trans. in part by Erling Eng (New York: Basic Books, 1966), pp. 4–11.

15. Cf. Hans Jonas, *The Phenomenon of Life* (Chicago: University of Chicago Press, 1966), pp. 145–49.

16. Indeed, as Merleau-Ponty points out (*Phenomenology of Perception,* pp. 225–35), the senses are lived as unified via a preobjective bodily synthesis, such that synesthesia is the rule more than the exception.

17. See, for example, Straus, *Phenomenological Psychology,* pp. 268–74.

18. See, for example, Michael Polanyi, *Knowing and Being,* ed. Marjorie Grene (Chicago: University of Chicago Press, 1969), pp. 138–58.

19. Ibid., pp. 147–48.

20. One of the deficiencies in Polanyi's account is his failure to elaborate upon the important functional and experiential differences between different elements in the "from" structure. For example, the role played in perception by extrinsic perceptual particulars is quite different from that of our body's kinesthesias or the fully tacit operations of our nervous system. Polanyi, for the most part, groups these together, paying but slight attention to the distinctions. However, I do agree with his point that at root all these examples manifest the same principle of from-to transitivity.

21. Polanyi, *Knowing and Being,* pp. 139–40.

22. Ibid., p. 139.

23. Ibid., p. 147; pp. 211–24.

24. Straus, *The Primary World of Senses,* pp. 233–36. Cf. Jonas, *The Phenomenon of Life,* pp. 152–56.

25. Straus, *The Primary World of Senses,* p. 198. As Heidegger points out, the pure theoretical perception thought to characterize scientific apprehension is in fact a derivative phenomenon. It arises only as a holding back from our usual concernful relations. See Martin Heidegger, *Being and Time,* trans. John Macquarrie and Edward Robinson (New York: Harper and Row, 1962), p. 89.

26. Paul Ricoeur, *Freedom and Nature: The Voluntary and the Involuntary,* trans. Erazim Kohák (Evanston, Ill.: Northwestern University Press, 1966), p. 210.

27. This is not to deny a certain body-awareness that ceaselessly accompanies activity. Ricoeur acknowledges that while primarily directing attention

to the desired goal, one maintains a "secondary, marginal consciousness" of one's own physical activity (*Freedom and Nature,* p. 216). We rely upon various kinesthesias in order to act successfully, continually adjusting the strength and direction of movement in response to these cues. Yet, as we have seen, these cues are employed in a subsidiary fashion. There is no need, and it would usually be disruptive, to explicitly thematize this body-sense.

28. See Heidegger, *Being and Time,* pp. 42n, 83, 88.

29. David Hume, *An Enquiry Concerning Human Understanding,* ed. Eric Steinberg (Indianapolis: Hackett Publishing, 1977), pp. 43–44.

30. Cf. Straus's similar point concerning the physicist in *The Primary World of Senses,* p. 110.

31. Merleau-Ponty, *Phenomenology of Perception,* p. 137.

32. Ibid., p. 94.

33. See Heidegger, *Being and Time,* pp. 172–79; and Robert C. Solomon, *The Passions* (Notre Dame, Ind.: University of Notre Dame Press, 1983).

34. Ricoeur, *Freedom and Nature,* p. 271.

35. Sartre, *Being and Nothingness,* p. 429.

36. Straus, *The Primary World of Senses,* pp. 379–85.

37. Jonas, *The Phenomenon of Life,* pp. 101–2.

38. See Merleau-Ponty, *Phenomenology of Perception,* pp. xvii, 137, 243.

39. Franz Brentano, *Psychology from an Empirical Standpoint,* ed. Oskar Kraus, trans. Antos C. Rancurello, D. B. Terrell, and Linda L. McAlister (London: Routledge and Kegan Paul, 1973), pp. 88–89.

40. Heidegger, in *Being and Time,* applied the term of "ecstasis" particularly to this projective nature of temporality (p. 377). However, in this area, as in others, he fails to develop the crucial role played by the lived body.

41. Ibid., p. 60.

42. Husserl, *Ideen 2,* p. 146.

43. Oliver Sacks, *The Man who Mistook his Wife for a Hat* (New York: Harper and Row, 1987), pp. 43–54.

44. Ibid., p. 49.

45. Merleau-Ponty, *The Visible and the Invisible,* pp. 140–42.

46. This phrase appeared in the French edition of Husserl's *Cartesian Meditations* (though the author came to expunge it from the German) and, along with similar wordings in *Ideen 2,* made an appreciable impact on Merleau-Ponty. He refers to it, for instance, in *The Visible and the Invisible,* p. 256, and in "The Philosopher and his Shadow," in *Signs,* trans. Richard C. McCleary (Evanston, Ill.: Northwestern University Press, 1964), pp. 166, 168.

47. Richard Zaner, *The Context of Self* (Athens: Ohio University Press, 1981), p. 45.

48. Zaner, drawing upon the work of Gurwitsch, calls the body a "contexture." That is, it is a system organized by a unifying principle or agency beyond its constituent parts, wherein each part gains its functional significance only by virtue of its place in the overall structure. The contexture is characterized by a tendency to complete and maintain its general coherence. See *The Context of Self,* pp. 77–82 and 93–99.

49. van den Berg, "The Human Body and the Significance of Human Movement," pp. 169–70.

50. Sigmund Freud, *Introductory Lectures on Psychoanalysis,* trans. James Strachey (New York: W. W. Norton, 1966), p. 347.

51. Ibid.

52. Sigmund Freud, *Three Essays on the Theory of Sexuality,* trans. James Strachey (New York: Basic Books, 1962), p. 106.

53. I am suggesting that an organ cannot simultaneously play a focal and background role relative to any one activity. However, because the corporeal field contains multiple sensorimotor gestalts, an organ may function as background to one activity and focus of another, and thereby be enveloped in both modes of disappearance. To use an earlier example, if I am tying knots in a string while intently gazing at a landscape, my fingers are forgotten in a twofold way. First, they are backgrounded vis-à-vis my dominant visual project. Second, they focally disappear within their own actional field as the means from which I manipulate the string.

54. Charles Sherrington, *The Integrative Action of the Nervous System* (New Haven, Conn.: Yale University Press, 1947), pp. 323–24.

55. Philip Kapleau, ed., *The Three Pillars of Zen* (Boston: Beacon Press, 1965), pp. 67–68.

56. While anything like a comprehensive phenomenological anatomy yet remains to be constructed, important works in this area have already appeared. For example, one can point to Erwin Straus's investigations concerning the significance of the upright posture and the phenomenological characteristics of the different senses, as included in the collection *Phenomenological Psychology,* or, in a more lighthearted vein, Richard M. Griffith's exploration of the existentialia of the foot in "Anthropodology: Man A-Foot," in *The Philosophy of the Body,* ed. Stuart F. Spicker (Chicago: Quadrangle Books, 1970), pp. 273–92.

57. Leibniz, "Monadology," in *Discourse on Metaphysics, Correspondence with Arnauld, Monadology,* trans. George R. Montgomery (La Salle, Ill.: Open Court, 1980), p. 267.

58. Gilbert Ryle, *The Concept of Mind* (New York: Barnes and Noble, 1949), pp. 25–61.

59. Polanyi, *Knowing and Being,* pp. 141–42.

60. See Wittgenstein's argument that to understand something is not to undergo an instantaneous mental event but to be able to successfully perform tasks. Ludwig Wittgenstein, *Philosophical Investigations,* trans. G. E. M. Anscombe (New York: Macmillan, 1953), pp. 53–61, 104–6 (remarks 138–55, 318–25).

61. Ricoeur, *Freedom and Nature,* p. 282.

62. As Edward S. Casey has explored, beneath our thematic memory of specific images and representations lies a pervasive "body memory" retaining abilities, habits, ways of experiencing the world. See *Remembering* (Bloomington: Indiana University Press, 1987), pp. 146–80.

63. Ricoeur, *Freedom and Nature,* pp. 285–86.

64. Heidegger, *Being and Time,* pp. 95–107.

65. Polanyi, *Knowing and Being,* p. 145.

66. Merleau-Ponty, *Phenomenology of Perception,* p. 143.

67. This process is intimately intertwined with that discussed in relation to skill acquisition, for the incorporation of a tool always involves the concurrent mastery of the skill whereby it is employed. The blind man incorporates not only the stick but a new sensorimotor schema.

68. Merleau-Ponty, *Phenomenology of Perception,* p. 143.

69. Don Ihde recognizes this same phenomenon under a different name: "I may describe these relations as *embodiment relations,* relations in which the machine displays some kind of partial transparency so that it itself does not become objectified or thematic, but is taken into my experiencing of what is other in the World" (*Technics and Praxis* [Dordrecht: D. Reidel, 1979], p. 8). This transparency is never complete; as Ihde points out, there is always an "echo focus" (p. 7), a subliminal awareness of the instrument at my body boundary. Moreover, especially at times of malfunction, the tool can become thematically central. (See chapter 3, below, for a fuller discussion of this principle and its application to bodily dysfunction.)

70*. A recognition of the close relationship between the body and its instruments has most frequently taken the form of likening the body itself to a tool or machine. Yet as Gabriel Marcel points out, such a model leads to difficulties. See *Metaphysical Journal,* trans. Bernard Wall (Chicago: Henry Regnery, 1952), p. 246. Cf. Merleau-Ponty, *The Structure of Behavior,* pp. 208–9. If our body were itself a tool, there would need to be a second, more primordial body that uses it, *ad infinitum.* Yet to terminate this regress by conceiving of the soul or mind as what wields the body-tool raises further problems. As Marcel notes, this attributes to the soul all the potentialities the body actualizes (perception, motility, expression, etc.), which would indeed make the soul into something like a second body. Moreover, by envisioning the body as a mere tool, we vitiate it of all its powers and animacy. This external, instrumental relation between mind and body fails to do justice to the unity of lived experience. Even Descartes, the most famous proponent of the body-as-machine, recognizes this when arguing that the mind is far more intimately conjoined to the body than is a pilot to his ship. The true relation between body and instrument, phenomenological rather than crudely materialistic in character, is only revealed when we reverse the analogy. It is not that the body is like a tool, but that the tool is like a second sort of body, incorporated into and extending our corporeal powers.

71*. Far from being a univocal phenomenon, technologies can manifest a range of different functional and experiential structures. Hence, my analysis, based primarily on the paradigm of the tool, is ultimately insufficient to do justice to the complexity of modern technology. In this extended footnote I will seek to suggest a way in which the categories of bodily disappearance can help articulate the essential features of differing sorts of technologies.

To this end I will utilize a scheme suggested by Ladislav Tondl. (See "On the Concept of 'Technology' and 'Technological Sciences,' " in *Contributions to a Philosophy of Technology*, ed. Frederich Rapp [Dordrecht: D. Reidel, 1974], pp. 10–11.) Tondl divides technology into three essential phases. First was the era of tools proper, such as axes, hammers and chisels, activated by muscle power. Second, came the invention of machines, a category that classically includes all devices powered by nonhuman energy sources. Originally relying on natural means such as animals, wind, and water, these later came to utilize a variety of mechanical engines. Human beings guide and control these machines but do not supply their motive force. Finally, in the third stage, there is the development of "automated machines." These use cybernetic principles of self-monitoring and self-regulation to perform themselves many of the control functions hitherto carried out by people.

Clearly, the body-instrument relation is quite different in these three phases of technology. As discussed, in the tool-phase the instrument in use can best be understood as incorporated within the body's focal disappearance. The human body wields and powers the tool. However, in the case of the machine it is more a question of the human body itself being placed into a background disappearance. The body, no longer supplying the direct force and pattern for the work, is relegated to a supporting role vis-à-vis many machine operations. The wind grinds grain that before was ground by hand. The factory makes furniture that before a human body fashioned, supplemented by its tools.

This background disappearance lies at the root of many of the favorable and unfavorable repercussions of industrialization. On the one hand, this back-grounding of the human body serves a liberating function, for machines can take over physically difficult or uninteresting work, leaving people free for more satisfying tasks. On the other hand, as machines increasingly usurp the labor process, unemployment can result, an extreme picture of the body put out of play. Furthermore, even when one's job is retained, its character may be markedly altered. Prior to the spread of industrialization the craft worker was intimately involved in many stages of the manufacturing process, so that the final product was the direct result of his or her skill and vision. This is often not the case with machine-dominated labor. Rather than being freed from uninteresting work, the factory laborer may find him or herself restricted to limited and repetitious tasks mandated by the process. The needs and rhythms of the machine rather than those of the human body control the work. This back-grounding of the body thus plays a crucial part in creating the alienated labor that Karl Marx describes as typical of industrial capitalism (see *The Economic and Philosophical Manuscripts of 1844*, ed. Dick J. Struik [New York: International Publishers, 1964], pp. 106–19).

In the machine phase this background disappearance is characterized primarily by the body's relegation to a supportive function. Bodies are still required to guide equipment operation, thereby supporting the needs of the machine. With the introduction of the self-regulating "automated machine" direct bodily involvement is even further reduced. The body is now backgrounded primarily because it has been put out of play. Instead of having to shovel coal for the furnace, one merely leaves the thermostat at the desired temperature. Whereas the pilot's vision and manual skill may once have guided a flight, the automata of the plane now accomplish it with little human assistance. The use of sensorimotor powers in the labor process becomes increasingly tangential in this automated age.

Moreover, this disappearance of the body often coincides with an experiential disappearance of the automaton itself. Albert Borgmann describes this process in reference to what he terms the "device paradigm" of modern technology (*Technology and the Character of Contemporary Life* [Chicago: University of Chicago Press, 1984], pp. 40–48). A "device," the central structure of modern technology, is that which provides the most of any commodity we seek (warmth, comfort, entertainment, etc.) while demanding the least amount of attention to its operation. For example, we expect our television to work with a flick of the wrist. Yet as Borgmann points out, precisely because the device makes no demands, it tends toward a form of concealment. Few know or care precisely the way a central heating plant functions, or a computer, or a telephone system. We do not need to, for we connect with such instruments only tangentially at the point of receiving their commodity. Thus, while tools conceal themselves through their incorporation within the body, these automata disappear by virtue of their distance from the body; their inner workings are hidden away from our direct perception and control. See Drew Leder, "The Rule of the Device: Borgmann's Philosophy of Technology," *Philosophy Today* 32 (1988): 17–29.

Ultimately, this disappearance of the body and automaton alike can bring about a sort of world-disappearance, a reduction of certain possibilities of encounter. As Borgmann argues, direct corporeal involvement with work created a context of social and natural relations, many of which have been removed by technological "disburdenment." When we still needed a woodstove, not a thermostat, to secure warmth, trees had to be felled, logs split, wood hauled. In Borgmann's words, "It provided for the entire family a regular and bodily engagement with the rhythm of the seasons that was woven together of the threat of cold and the solace of warmth, the smell of wood smoke, the exertion of sawing and of carrying, the teaching of skills, and the fidelity to daily tasks" (p. 42). Though the central heating plant is surely convenient, it cannot provide us with a rich context for living. Again, technology presents a two-edged sword; automata can efface drudgery, but they can also vitiate our engagements with the world.

72*. When incorporating a tool, one's concurrent incorporation by it may have a series of unanticipated results. As Ihde notes, every instrument imposes an "amplification-reduction" structure on one's natural capacities (*Technics and Praxis,* pp. 9–10, 21–26). The telephone, while allowing communication through its amplification of voice, in other ways yields a reduced encounter devoid of direct sight and touch. As a result of such transformations, each technology provides a "telic inclination" toward certain modified modes of interaction (pp. 42–44). I speak differently on the phone than I do in person, just as this work has been influenced by its creation on a computer, not through the medium of typewriter or pen. See Michael Heim, *Electric Language: A Philosophical Study of Word Processing* (New Haven, Conn.: Yale University Press, 1987).

73. Elaine Scarry, *The Body in Pain* (New York: Oxford University Press, 1985), pp. 38–39.

Chapter Two: The Recessive Body

1. In the *Phenomenology of Perception,* Merleau-Ponty does, at certain points, acknowledge the radical impersonality of our organismic existence (pp. 83–85), of a natural life, a birth and death that outstrips the personal "I" (pp. 331, 364). Yet, he never fully develops the far-reaching implications of such themes. They are subordinated to discussions of perception and motility.

2. F. J. J. Buytendijk, *Prolegomena to an Anthropological Physiology* (Pittsburgh: Duquesne University Press, 1974).

3. In the original proposal of this classification by Sherrington, the "interoceptive" field was equated solely with the digestive surface (*Integrative Action,* p. 317). In common usage, it has since expanded to include all visceral sensation. The term *interoceptor* is often used to refer to all forms of visceral receptor, not excluding those which initiate strictly unconscious homeostatic circuits. However, in my employment, "interoception" refers solely to what is capable of entering conscious experience.

4. Neurophysiologists usually attribute this to the relative paucity of visceral afferent nerves, as well as to their intrinsic and distributional characteristics.

5. Arthur C. Guyton, *Textbook of Medical Physiology,* 7th ed. (Philadelphia: W. B. Saunders, 1986), p. 598.

6. Other physiological factors, too extensive to treat at length, contribute to the ambiguous spatiality of visceral events. For example, an initially localized pain can depolarize surrounding nerve roots, leading to a generalization. Conversely, when the parietal membrane adjoining the viscus becomes involved, pain can suddenly and sharply localize. As a result of such factors a disease such as appendicitis often proceeds through two or three different experiential stages in which the quality and distribution of pain transform.

7. Ricoeur, *Freedom and Nature,* p. 412.

8. Guyton, *Medical Physiology,* p. 599. It is worth noting that while the parenchyma of the liver is insensitive, this is not true of the liver capsule or bile ducts; similarly, the bronchi and parietal pleura of the lung are sensitive.

9. Cf. Zaner's discussion of the body as "hidden presence" in *The Context of Self,* pp. 53–54.

10*. The lived experience of the inner body may be better expressed by certain non-Western medicines and cosmologies than by the anatomical descriptions of the West. Chinese Taoists picture the viscera as centers along greater and lesser pathways for the circulation of *ch'i,* a blood/breath energy (see chapter 6, below). Similarly, Buddhists envision a "subtle body" as well as a physical, with *chakras,* nodes through which *prana,* a subtle breath, flows. Such schemas are meant to have not only explanatory but phenomenological power, charting experiences open to the ordinary person or to those who engage in spiritual practices. These energic portrayals may capture the subtle and shifting quality of inner experience better than an image of fixed, massy organs.

11. Michel Foucault, *The Birth of the Clinic,* trans. A. M. Sheridan Smith (New York: Vintage Books, 1975), p. 166.

12. Straus, *The Primary World of Senses,* pp. 231–71.

13. Ibid., pp. 264–66.

14. Cf. Zaner on the "alien presence" of the body, in *The Context of Self,* pp. 54–55.

15. Ricoeur, *Freedom and Nature,* p. 418.

16. *The Passions of the Soul,* in *The Philosophical Works of Descartes,* 2 vols., ed. Elizabeth Haldane and G. R. T. Ross (Cambridge: Cambridge University Press, 1985), 1: 339.

17. Aristotle, *De Anima,* in *The Basic Works of Aristotle,* ed. Richard McKeon (New York: Random House, 1941), pp. 555, 561.

18. This is not to deny that visceral organs have a limited plasticity and ability to exchange functions. For example, lung and kidney cooporate to regulate acid-base metabolism, and when one organ is partially disabled the other will modify its function in the attempt to restore homeostasis.

19. Buytendijk, *Prolegomena,* p. 135.

20. As Zaner notes, the own-body is not simply that which is mine; I also *belong to it* (*The Context of Self,* p. 52).

21. Buytendijk, *Prolegomena,* p. 295.

22. Merleau-Ponty, *Phenomenology of Perception,* p. 94.

23. Lewis Thomas, *The Lives of a Cell* (New York: Bantam Books, 1974), p. 78.

24. See Sherrington, *Integrative Action,* pp. 324–28, on the importance of distance receptors in permitting appropriate anticipatory reactions on the part of the animal.

25. Ibid., p. 332.

26. Because of the possibility of intentional control we have over breathing, and its immediate shifts in response to emotion, Buytendijk writes that breathing is "based in existence more than any other physiological function" (*Prolegomena,* p. 285).

27. On medicine as hermeneutic enterprise, see Stephen L. Daniel, "The Patient as Text: A Model of Clinical Hermeneutics," *Theoretical Medicine* 7 (1986): 195–210; and Drew Leder, "Clinical Interpretation: The Hermeneutics of Medicine," *Theoretical Medicine,* forthcoming.

28. Quoted in Kim Chernin, *The Obsession* (New York: Harper and Row, 1981), p. 4.

29. As Descartes notes in a letter to Elizabeth, recommending psychological remedies for her ills: "The soul guides the spirits into the places where they can be useful or harmful; however, it does not do this by a direct volition, but only by willing or thinking about something else. For our body is so constructed that certain of its motions follow naturally upon certain thoughts: as we see that blushes accompany shame, tears compassions, and laughter joy" (*Philosophical*

Letters, trans. and ed. Anthony Kenny [Minneapolis: University of Minnesota Press, 1970], p. 153, cf. pp. 161–63). It is interesting that, while Cartesian metaphysics is at the root of our current mechanistic medicine (see chapter 5, below), Descartes himself was an early "holistic practitioner," emphasizing to Elizabeth the importance of diet, exercise, and above all, proper thinking, in treating her malady.

30. Neal E. Miller, "Biofeedback and Visceral Learning," in *Biofeedback and Self-Control 1977/78,* ed. Johann Stoyva et al. (New York: Aldine Publishing Company, 1979), pp. 421–52.

31. Ibid., pp. 426–28. Cf. Jasper Brener, "Sensory and Perceptual Determinants of Voluntary Visceral Control," in *Biofeedback: Theory and Research,* ed. Gary E. Schwartz and Jackson Beatty (New York: Academic Press, 1977), pp. 29–66.

32. John V. Basmajian, ed., *Biofeedback: Principles and Practice for Clinicians,* 3d ed. (Baltimore: Williams and Wilkins, 1989); and Leonard White and Bernard Tursky, eds., *Clinical Biofeedback: Efficacy and Mechanisms* (New York: Guilford Press, 1982).

33. See, for example, Elmer Green and Alyce Green, *Beyond Biofeedback* (San Francisco: Delacorte Press, 1977); and Patricia Norris, "Biofeedback, Voluntary Control, and Human Potential," *Biofeedback and Self-Regulation* 11 (1986): 1–20.

34. See, for example, Merleau-Ponty, *Phenomenology of Perception,* pp. 154–73, esp. 168, and pp. 380–81.

35*. This sense of a visceral root of the unconscious is, to a degree, present in Freud. The "ego" is specifically identified with a perceptual consciousness ("the system *Pcpt.-Cs.*") that arises from the body surface and its interaction with the outer world (Sigmund Freud, *The Ego and the Id,* ed. James Strachey, trans. Joan Riviere [New York, W. W. Norton, 1960], pp. 9–17). Conversely, instincts are "the representatives of all the forces originating in the interior of the body and transmitted to the mental apparatus" (Sigmund Freud, *Beyond the Pleasure Principle,* trans. and ed. James Strachey [New York, W. W. Norton, 1961]). Consciousness, as associated with a limited corporeal layer—what I have termed the surface, ecstatic body—has only an indirect awareness of and control over impulses from the deeper soma.

36. See Zaner, *The Context of Self,* pp. 95–96, on the complex range of variation concerning the degree of personal awareness and control exerted over different bodily functions. He calls attention to the intermediate states of the complemental series whose poles we have articulated.

37. As Merleau-Ponty suggests, even perception itself has a radically anonymous and impersonal aspect. "Each sensation, being strictly speaking, the first, last and only one of its kind, is a birth and a death. The subject who experiences it begins and ends with it, and as he can neither precede nor survive himself, sensation necessarily appears to itself in a setting of generality, its origin is anterior to myself, it arises from *sensibility* which has preceded it and which will outlive it, just as my birth and death belong to a natality and a mortality which are anonymous" (*Phenomenology of Perception,* p. 216). While I have empha-

sized the crucial divergence of ecstatic and recessive modes, such statements help to point out their intimate intertwining.

38. Straus, *The Primary World of Senses,* p. 285.

39. Merleau-Ponty, *Phenomenology of Perception,* p. 163.

40. This is not to claim that the temporal series of sleeping-waking is strictly equivalent to that of body surface-depth; the waking body also includes visceral depths within it. Nevertheless, we might say that wakefulness is most characterized by the eruption of ecstasis, the body asleep, by its recessive retreat. (The same impure equivalence marks the next series to be discussed, that of the prenatal versus the adult body.)

41. The dreaming state is not only an interweaving of aspects of the sleeping and waking body but produces yet another "imaginal" body with its own idiosyncratic features. An exploration of this three-sided corporeality of the dreaming subject would make an interesting study, but one that I will not attempt here. See Arnold Mindell, *Working with the Dreaming Body* (Boston: Routledge and Kegan Paul, 1985).

42. Ricoeur, *Freedom and Nature,* p. 433.

43. Merleau-Ponty, *Phenomenology of Perception,* p. 347; also see pp. 215–16, 331, 363–64, 407, 428.

44. Margaret S. Mahler, Fred Pine, and Anni Bergman, *The Psychological Birth of the Human Infant* (New York: Basic Books, 1975), esp. pp. 41–64.

45. David Winnicott, *The Family and Individual Development* (London: Tavistock Publications, 1965), p. 17.

46. See Jacques Lacan, "The mirror stage as formative of the function of the I," in *Ecrits,* trans. Alan Sheridan (New York: W. W. Norton, 1977), pp. 1–7; and Maurice Merleau-Ponty, "The Child's Relations with Others," in *The Primacy of Perception,* ed. James M. Edie (Evanston, Ill.: Northwestern University Press, 1964), pp. 96–155., esp. pp. 113–41.

47. Merleau-Ponty, *The Primacy of Perception,* pp. 12–42.

48. Merleau-Ponty, *The Visible and the Invisible,* p. 183. Hereafter, in this section, all references will be cited in parentheses within the text using the abbreviation *VI* and the page number.

49. Gary Brent Madison, *The Phenomenology of Merleau-Ponty* (Athens: Ohio University Press, 1981).

50. On the concept of "identity-within-difference," and for a treatment of the notion of "flesh" upon which I here draw, see Martin Dillon, "Merleau-Ponty and the Reversibility Thesis," *Man and World* 16 (1983): 365–88. This material is also to be found in the book by M. C. Dillon, *Merleau-Ponty's Ontology* (Bloomington: Indiana University Press, 1988), pp. 153–76.

51. *The Random House Dictionary of the English Language: College Edition,* ed. Laurence Urdang (New York: Random House, 1968).

52*. The notion of "flesh and blood" is here meant to serve as a description of lived experience and our relation to the life-world. Unlike Merleau-Ponty I am not proposing it as an ontological notion, though I believe it has ontological ramifications. To work these out would require addressing questions of the following sort: Does the inanimate and the purely vegetative world partake of both flesh and blood? In what sense? Could one or the other term of this relation be more primary? If not, does this threaten us with a new dualism? Are "flesh" and "blood" not two manifestations arising from a common ground? Such ontological explorations would, however, take us beyond the boundaries of the current project.

53. For explanations and imaginative treatments of this principle, see Lewis Thomas's *The Lives of a Cell*, and Lynn Margulis and Dorion Sagan, *Microcosmos: Four Billion Years of Evolution from our Microbial Ancestors* (New York: Summit Books, 1986).

54. As Straus writes: "[The sleeper] has, in fact, not withdrawn his interest from the world; rather, in lying down and sleeping he gives himself completely to the world. He gives up his stance which 'opposes' and confronts the world. Thus, he can no longer freely relate to the world and therefore no longer delimit and claim that which is his own" (*The Primary World of Senses*, p. 284).

55. See Jonas, *The Phenomenon of Life*, pp. 99–107, and Sherrington, *Integrative Action*, pp. 324–28.

56*. The threatening nature of the "look" Sartre describes (pp. 340–400) can be understood in this biological context. For Sartre, insofar as I am perceiving subject I turn the Other into an object, and hence a wrestling for power ensues (see chapter 3, below). The root of the threat involved is clear on an animal level; encountering another living thing, I may be the eater, but I am also vulnerable to being eaten. Whether the body assumes a subject or object role can literally be a matter of life and death in the animal kingdom.

It is, however, worth noting that life preserves itself not only through the destruction of, but a mutuality with, other life. My exhaled carbon dioxide is food to the plants while their oxygen sustains me. As ecologists are detailing, the biosphere maintains itself largely through such complementary exchanges. For a discussion of this principle and its relation to Merleau-Pontian phenomenology see David Abram, "The Perceptual Implications of Gaia," *The Ecologist* 15 (1985): 96–103.

57*. In "Eye and Mind," the last work published in his lifetime, Merleau-Ponty writes, "It can be said that a human is born at the instant when something that was only virtually visible, inside the mother's body, becomes at one and the same time visible for itself and for us" (*The Primacy of Perception*, pp. 167–68). However, this is but a brief reference designed to explicate the birth of perception in the painter. Indeed, Merleau-Ponty often uses sexual and birth imagery in his discussions of perception. It is characterized as a mutual interpenetration of subject and object, or a "natal bond with the world" (*VI*, 32). Perceptual intersubjectivity comes to be when "the other is born in the body (of the other)" and there is a "coupling of the bodies" (*VI*, 233). Merleau-Ponty's language always bears a suggestion of the visceral chiasm that perception mirrors and sublimates. Yet he rarely engages the visceral as a phenomenon in its own right. When, for example, he writes in *The Visible and the Invisible* of the embryo, it is merely as a preliminary stage for the perceiving subject, a set of unemployed circuits preparing for the advent of vision (*VI*, 147, 233–34).

58*. Because of their bodily involvement in the reproductive cycle through hormonal shifts, menstruation, and pregnancy, women may tend to have a greater awareness of this visceral dimension of embodiment and intersubjectivity than do men. It is probably no coincidence that this dimension has been neglected by *male* philosophers. For a discussion of the lived body in pregnancy, see Iris Young, "Pregnant Embodiment: Subjectivity and Alienation," *The Journal of Medicine and Philosophy* 9 (1984): 45–62.

59. See Wing-Tsit Chan, ed., *A Sourcebook in Chinese Philosophy* (Princeton, N.J.: Princeton University Press, 1963), p. 412.

Chapter Three: The Dys-appearing Body

1. Guyton, *Medical Physiology*, p. 593.

2. See, for example, Tolstoy's "The Death of Ivan Ilych," for a vivid expression of the way pain, disease, and impending death can expose the hollowness at the heart of one's world. A bridge game that once brought excitement, judicial duties which once seemed quite important, are now exposed in their absurdity, their impotence to ward off present pain and a dreaded future. However, as the finale of the story suggests, this undermining of habitual concerns can prepare the way for the advent of novel meanings; Ivan is forced by suffering to confront his life and death authentically for the first time.

3. Scarry, *The Body in Pain,* p. 4.

4. John Updike, "Pain," *The New Republic,* 26 December 1983, p. 34.

5. See David Bakan, *Disease, Pain, and Sacrifice* (Boston: Beacon Press, 1971), p. 66.

6. F. J. J. Buytendijk, *Pain: Its Modes and Functions,* trans. Eda O'Shiel (Chicago: University of Chicago Press, 1962), p. 25.

7. Scarry, *The Body in Pain,* p. 35.

8. Emily Dickinson, *The Complete Poems of Emily Dickinson,* ed. Thomas H. Johnson (Boston: Little, Brown and Company, 1960), pp. 323–24.

9. Drew Leder, "Toward a Phenomenology of Pain," *Review of Existential Psychology and Psychiatry* 19 (1984–85): 255–66.

10. Cf. Zaner, *The Context of Self,* pp. 54–55.

11. Thus, for Descartes it is experiences such as pain, hunger, and thirst that show that the mind does not merely reside in the body like a pilot in a ship but is closely united with it. *Meditations,* in *The Philosophical Works of Descartes,* 2 vols., ed. Elizabeth Haldane and G. R. T. Ross (Cambridge: Cambridge University Press, 1911) 1:192.

12. J. C. White and W. H. Sweet, *Pain: Its Mechanisms and Neurosurgical Control* (Springfield, Ill.: Charles C. Thomas, 1955), p. 108. As cited in Bakan, *Disease, Pain, and Sacrifice,* pp. 74–75.

13. See Buytendijk, *Pain,* p. 26. It is not arbitrary that I choose to focus on instances where pain is involuntary, as with injury or disease. The aversive quality of pain and its role as a signal of physiological distress assure that in most cases pain will be an undesired occurrence. However, there are many counterexamples: e.g., the athlete referred to in the text, or, most famously, the masochist. Because pain is not simply an objective but an existential event, it is

susceptible to a wide range of differing interpretations depending on the life-world context in which it unfolds.

14. Bakan, *Disease, Pain, and Sacrifice,* p. 77.

15. Drew Leder, "Medicine and Paradigms of Embodiment," *The Journal of Medicine and Philosophy* 9 (1984): 33. Cf. Buytendijk, *Prolegomena,* p. 61.

16. Herbert Plügge, "Man and His Body," trans. Erling Eng, in *The Philosophy of the Body,* ed. Stuart F. Spicker (Chicago: Quadrangle Books, 1970), pp. 293–311. From Herbert Plügge, *Der Mensch und sein Leib* (Tubingen: Max Niemeyer Verlag, 1967), pp. 34–42, 57–68.

17. Sartre, *Being and Nothingness,* p. 438.

18. The epistemic significance of pain can be traced back to early childhood. Freud, among others, has suggested that pain plays an important part in forming the infant's body image and delineating the body-world division. See Sigmund Freud, *Civilization and its Discontents,* trans. and ed. James Strachey (New York: W. W. Norton, 1961), p. 14. Elsewhere he writes that "the way in which we gain new knowledge of our organs during painful illnesses is perhaps a model of the way by which in general we arrive at the idea of our body" (*The Ego and the Id,* pp. 15–16).

19. Bakan, *Pain, Disease, and Sacrifice,* pp. 57–58.

20. Thomas S. Szasz, *Pain and Pleasure* (New York: Basic Books, 1957), p. 203.

21*. As Hans-Georg Gadamer notes, the question of pragmatic application is integral to the hermeneutic project as a whole (*Truth and Method* [New York: Crossroad, 1975], pp. 274–305). The interpreter strives to understand a text partially to determine its applicability to his or her own situation. We seek to know in order to do, and our possibilities of doing help determine our objects and modes of knowing. Hence, what I term the *hermeneutic* and *pragmatic* moments are not ultimately separate categories but are closely interwoven and interdependent.

Gadamer refers to legal hermeneutics to exemplify this centrality of application to understanding. An examination of medical hermeneutics provides another striking illustration. The physician seeks to understand the patient's signs and symptoms in order to arrive at an efficacious treatment. Diagnosis and therapy, understanding and praxis, are inseparably linked. See Leder, "Clinical Interpretation."

22. See Mary C. Rawlinson, "Medicine's Discourse and the Practice of Medicine," and Edmund D. Pellegrino, "Being Ill and Being Healed," in *The Humanity of the Ill,* ed. Victor Kestenbaum (Knoxville: University of Tennessee Press, 1982), pp. 69–95 and 157–66; J. H. van den Berg, *The Psychology of the Sickbed* (Pittsburgh: Duquesne University Press, 1966); and Herbert Plügge, *Wohlbefinden und Missbefinden* (Tubingen: Max Niemeyer Verlag, 1962).

23. See, for example, H. Tristram Engelhardt, Jr., "The Concepts of Health and Disease," in *Evaluation and Explanation in the Biomedical Sciences,* vol. 1, ed. H. Tristram Engelhardt, Jr. and Stuart F. Spicker (Dordrecht: D. Reidel, 1975), pp. 125–41. This and many other relevant articles are included in Arthur

L. Caplan, H. Tristram Engelhardt, Jr., and James J. McCartney, eds., *Concepts of Health and Disease* (Reading, Mass.: Addison-Wesley Publishing Co., 1981).

24. See, for example, H. Tristram Engelhardt, Jr., "Illnesses, Diseases, and Sicknesses," in *The Humanity of the Ill,* ed. Victor Kestenbaum, pp. 142–56; Eric Cassell, *The Healer's Art* (Cambridge: MIT Press, 1985); and Sartre, *Being and Nothingness,* pp. 441–45, 456–58.

25. Buytendijk, *Prolegomena,* p. 62.

26. van den Berg, *Psychology of the Sickbed,* p. 26.

27. Plügge, *Wohlbefinden und Missbefinden,* pp. 129-35.

28. Ibid., p. 129.

29. H. Tristram Engelhardt, Jr., "Human Well-Being and Medicine: Some Basic Value-Judgments in the Biomedical Sciences," in *Science, Ethics and Medicine,* ed. H. Tristram Engelhardt, Jr., and Daniel Callahan (Hastings: Institute of Society, Ethics and the Life Sciences, 1976), pp. 120–39.

30. Plügge, *Wohlbefinden und Missbefinden,* pp. 91–106.

31. H. Plügge and R. Kohn, "Wohlbefinden und Missbefinden," in *Psyche* (1958): 40. As cited in Buytendijk, *Prolegomena,* p. 285.

32. Heidegger, *Being and Time,* pp. 279–311.

33. Ricoeur, *Freedom and Nature,* pp. 85–134.

34. Leo Tolstoy, *The Death of Ivan Ilych and Other Stories* (New York: The New American Library, 1960), p. 134.

35. Heidegger, *Being and Time,* pp. 95–107.

36. Ibid., p. 103.

37. See Plügge, *Wohlbefinden und Missbefinden,* pp. 94–95.

38. Michael Polanyi, *Personal Knowledge* (Chicago: University of Chicago Press, 1958), p. 56.

39. On this point, see Jonas, *The Phenomenon of Life,* pp. 7–37; Zaner, *The Context of Self,* p. 55; Leder, "Toward a Phenomenology of Pain," and Scarry, *The Body in Pain,* pp. 48–49.

40. Merleau-Ponty, *Phenomenology of Perception,* pp. 149–50.

41. G. W. F. Hegel, *Hegel's Philosophy of Nature,* vol. 3, trans. Michael John Perry (New York: Humanities Press, 1970), p. 193.

42. Ibid., p. 194.

43. Young, "Pregnant Embodiment," p. 49. See Merleau-Ponty, *Phenomenology of Perception,* p. 82, for the notion of the "habit-body" versus the "body at this moment."

44. Young, "Pregnant Embodiment," p. 56.

45. See, for example, Richard W. Wertz and Dorothy C. Wertz, *Lying In: A History of Childbirth in America* (New York: Schocken Books, 1979).

46. Sally Gadow, "Body and Self: A Dialectic," in *The Humanity of the Ill,* ed. Victor Kestenbaum (Knoxville: University of Tennessee Press, 1982), pp. 92–99.

47. Young, "Pregnant Embodiment," pp. 50–54.

48. One might argue that the emotional and existential power of such moments is matched by certain forms of bodily delight: for example, the intensity of sexual satisfaction or athletic accomplishment. I would not deny that this may at

times be true. However, as previously mentioned, the pleasurable tends to be more outward-focused and less demanding of interpretive reflection than times of corporeal dysfunction. It is true that the search for pleasure or success may come to dominate body awareness. One thinks of the frustrated lover consumed with lust or the athlete ceaselessly working to build up the body. Yet this merely confirms the power of dys-appearance; at such times, it is the problematic and as-yet-unfulfilled nature of bodily intention that brings the physical to prominence.

49. Jacques Lacan, *Ecrits,* pp. 1–7. Cf. Merleau-Ponty, *The Primacy of Perception,* pp. 136–38.

50. Sartre, *Being and Nothingness,* p. 434.

51. Ibid., pp. 436–40.

52. Ibid., p. 443.

53. Ibid., p. 461.

54. Ibid., p. 462.

55. Ibid., pp. 462–63.

56. Ibid., pp. 347–50.

57. Zaner, *The Context of Self,* pp. 47–66.

58. van den Berg, "The Human Body and the Significance of Human Movement," p. 175.

59. Merleau-Ponty, *Phenomenology of Perception,* p. 354.

60. Zaner, *The Context of Self,* p. 202.

61. Merleau-Ponty, *Phenomenology of Perception,* p. 352.

62. Anthropological studies reveal that the personal body is always already a social body, informed by the habits, expressions, ways of seeing and acting indigenous to the culture. See, for example, John Blacking, ed., *Anthropology of the Body* (New York: Academic Press, 1978); and Mary Douglas, *Natural Symbols* (New York: Panther Books, 1970).

63. Merleau-Ponty, *Phenomenology of Perception,* p. 361.

64. This is not to imply that it is only my physical body understood in a restricted sense that dys-appears at such times. In the face of a hostile gaze I may become aware of beliefs I hold which the Other might condemn, or a questionable past I now must conceal. Self-consciousness is heightened in a generalized fashion with this breakdown of mutuality.

65. van den Berg, "The Human Body and the Significance of Human Movement," p. 181.

66. Ibid., p. 182.

67. Michel Foucault, *Discipline and Punish,* trans. Alan Sheridan (New York: Vintage Books, 1979), p. 25.

68. Ibid., p. 26.

69. Simone de Beauvoir, *The Second Sex* (New York: Vintage Books, 1974).

70*. In this case as well, social dys-appearance can intertwine with dis-ability on the personal level. Young cites a typically "feminine" style of bodily comportment seen in contemporary society. There is a tendency not to bring the entire body into play, as in "throwing like a girl"; to have a closed gait and body stance; to underestimate physical strength and ability; to timid and reactive, rather than active, movement. As Young argues, this comportment is usually not related to biological incapacity and cannot fully be explained by lack of training. It can be understood in reference to the bodily objectification de Beauvoir describes. If one originally experiences one's body as given over to the Other's gaze, it will not be fully lived in a style of motoric transcendence. The body is then experienced as positioned in space, as much as its active constitutor, an object to be tended rather than fully employed, protected from others rather than opening onto the world. A restricted style of bodily usage results. See Iris Young, "Throwing Like a Girl: A Phenomenology of Feminine Bodily Comportment, Motility and Spatiality," *Human Studies* 3 (1980): 137–56.

71. Scarry, *The Body in Pain,* pp. 27–59.

72. Susan Bordo, "Anorexia Nervosa: Psychopathology as the Crystallization of Culture," *The Philosophical Forum* 17 (1985–86): 73–104.

Chapter Four: The Immaterial Body

1. For a discussion of the phenomenological significance of the Necker cube, see Don Ihde, *Experimental Phenomenology* (New York: G. P. Putnam's Sons, 1977), pp. 91–108.

2. However, as discussed in chapter 1, at any given time the corporeal field can contain within it multiple attentional and actional gestalts, such that an organ may function as background to one activity while being the focus of another. My ears, for example, are background relative to driving a car but play a focal role in simultaneously listening to the radio. My point is simply that the same organ cannot be both focus and background relative to any single action; more than one diagram would be needed to map the differing gestalt relations operative in a multi-involved body.

3. Merleau-Ponty, *Phenomenology of Perception,* pp. 3–63.

4. Descartes, *Letters,* pp. 119–20.

5. Descartes, *Philosophical Works* (Haldane and Ross), 1: 345. (Hereafter all references will be cited in the text using the abbreviation "HR" and the volume number.)

6. Descartes, *Letters,* p. 139.

7. Descartes, HR 2: 255.

8. For a discussion of this doctrine and, more generally, of Descartes's conflicting accounts concerning the mind-body union, see Ruth Mattern, "Descartes's Correspondence with Elizabeth: Concerning Both the Union and Distinction of Mind and Body," in *Descartes: Critical and Interpretive Studies,* ed. Michael Hooker (Baltimore: Johns Hopkins University Press, 1978), pp. 212–22.

9. Descartes, "Passions," HR 1: 345.

10. Ibid.

11. Descartes, *Letters,* p. 70.

12. Ibid., p. 71.

13. Descartes, "Reply to the Fifth Set of Objections," HR 2: 210.

14. Descartes, HR 1: 289.

15. Descartes, "Passions," HR 1: 345.

16. Ibid., p. 350.

17. Descartes, *The Principles of Philosophy,* HR 1: 293. Also see *Meditations,* HR 1: 196.

18. Descartes, "Principles," HR 1: 293.

19. Descartes, *Letters,* p. 38.

20. Straus, *The Primary World of Senses,* p. 158.

21. Warren Gorman, *Body Image and the Image of the Brain* (St. Louis: Warren H. Green, 1969), p. 249.

22. Aristotle, *De Partibus Animalium,* in *The Works of Aristotle,* ed. J. A. Smith and W. D. Ross (London: Oxford University Press, 1912), 5: 652b. 3–8.

23. Freud, *Beyond the Pleasure Principle,* p. 21.

24. Polanyi, *Knowing and Being,* p. 147.

25. Merleau-Ponty, *The Visible and the Invisible,* p. 261.

26. Descartes, *Principles,* HR 1: 240.

27. Cf. Richard Rorty, *Philosophy and the Mirror of Nature* (Princeton, N.J.: Princeton University Press, 1979), p. 53.

28. Descartes, HR 1: 153.

29. Ibid., p. 222.

30. Cf. Anthony Kenny, *Descartes: A Study of His Philosophy* (New York: Random House, 1968), pp. 68–69.

31. Rorty, *Mirror of Nature,* p. 50.

32. See, for example, Descartes, *Arguments Demonstrating the Existence of God,* HR 2: 52; *Meditations,* HR 1: 190; and *Principles,* HR 1: 266.

33. Jonas, *The Phenomenon of Life,* p. 135, and Rorty, *Mirror of Nature,* pp. 38–39. Rorty comments that it is fruitless to ask what linguistic, economic, or idle reasons stand behind this development of a visual metaphor for knowledge. In Jonas's piece we find the response; far from being arbitrary, such an analogy is naturally suggested by the intrinsic phenomenal properties of vision.

34. Plato *Republic* 533d, in *The Collected Dialogues,* ed. Edith Hamilton and Huntington Cairns (Princeton, N.J.: Princeton University Press, 1961), p. 765. Also cf. pp. 750 (518c) and 743–44 (508a–e).

35. Descartes, *Letters,* p. 67.

36. As Descartes writes, "I term that clear which is present and apparent to an attentive mind, in the same way as we assert that we see objects clearly when, being present to the regarding eye, they operate upon it with sufficient strength" (*Principles,* HR 1: 237).

37. Rorty, *Mirror of Nature,* p. 45.

38. Jonas, *The Phenomenon of Life,* pp. 135–56.

39. Straus, *Phenomenological Psychology,* pp. 4–21, and *The Primary World of Senses,* pp. 367–79.

40. Descartes, *The Philosophical Writings of Descartes,* trans. John Cottingham, Robert Stoothoff, and Dugald Murdoch (Cambridge: Cambridge University Press, 1985), 1: 152.

41. Jonas, *The Phenomenon of Life,* pp. 145–49.

42. Ibid., p. 147.

43. Descartes, *Meditations,* HR 1: 188.

44. Descartes, *Principles,* HR 1: 238.

45. Descartes acknowledges this tension but does not think it exposes a fundamental problem in his thinking. As he writes in a letter to Gibieuf:

I do not see any difficulty in allowing on the one hand that the faculties of imagination and sensation belong to the soul, because they are species of thoughts, and on the other hand that they belong to the soul only as joined to the body, because they are kinds of thoughts without which one can conceive the soul entirely pure. (*Letters,* pp. 125–26)

46. Descartes, HR 1: 39.

47. Ibid., p. 186. This position, advanced prior to the proof of the existence of any body whatsoever, is necessarily couched as a hypothesis. However, it seems an accurate reflection of Descartes's final view.

48. Descartes, *Reply to the Fifth Set of Objections,* HR 2: 212.

49. Descartes, *Letters,* p. 66.

50. Ibid., p. 112.

51. Ibid., p. 134. Cf. pp. 72, 76, 148, 231.

52. Descartes, *Meditations,* HR 1: 185–86.

53. Descartes, *Letters,* pp. 105–6, 141.

54. Rorty, *Mirror of Nature,* pp. 47–51.

55. Wallace I. Matson, "Why Isn't the Mind-Body Problem Ancient?" in *Mind, Matter and Method: Essays in Philosophy and Science in Honor of Herbert Feigl,* ed. Paul Feyerabend and Grover Maxwell (Minneapolis: University of Minnesota Press, 1966), p. 101.

56. Plato *Phaedo* 66a, in *Collected Dialogues,* p. 48.

57. See, for example, Allan Paivia, *Imagery and Verbal Processes* (New York: Holt, Rinehart and Winston, 1971).

58. Descartes, *Letters,* p. 112.

59. Descartes, *Principles,* HR 1: 252.

60. Paivia, *Imagery and Verbal Processes,* pp. 16–18, 27.

61. Sartre, *Being and Nothingness,* p. 434.

62. Susanne Langer, *Philosophy in a New Key* (Cambridge: Harvard University Press, 1942), p. 75. Cf. Straus, *The Primary World of Senses,* pp. 152–53.

63. Bertrand Russell, *Philosophy* (New York: W. W. Norton, 1927), p. 44. (As cited in Langer, *Philosophy in a New Key,* p. 75.)

64. See Eric A. Havelock, "The Orality of Socrates and the Literacy of Plato: With Some Reflections on the Historical Origins of Moral Philosophy in Europe," in *New Essays on Socrates,* ed. Eugene Kelly (Washington D.C.: University Press of America, 1985), pp. 90–91.

65. David Abram, "The Consequences of Literacy; Reflections in the Shadow of Plato's *Phaedrus,*" State University of New York at Stony Brook, 1986, typescript. I am indebted to the author for first drawing to my attention the importance of literacy relative to the notion of mind.

66*. Eric A Havelock, *Preface to Plato* (Cambridge: Harvard University Press, Belknap Press, 1963), esp. pp. 197–213, 254–75. According to Havelock, the mnemonic necessities and modes of transmission to which an oral culture is tied encourage the use of highly imagistic and concrete language, along with an almost hypnotic identification of listener with speaker. Writing, on the other hand, permits the elaboration of abstract terms, the thematization of concepts as objects in themselves, the sense of a separate and critical thinker—leading to the emergence of the "intellect" as we now know it.

67. This is not to deny the crucial import of other phenomena in shaping Plato's doctrines; most importantly that of mathematics and of moral/spiritual intuitions.

68. For a landmark discussion of this point, see Wittgenstein's argument against the possibility of a private language in *Philosophical Investigations,* pp. 88–112 (remarks 241–352).

69. See, for example, Edmund Jacobson, "Electrical Measurements in Neuromuscular States During Mental Activities," in *American Journal of Physiology* 97 (1931): 200–209. This and other relevant articles are reprinted in *Thinking: Studies of Covert Language Processes,* ed. F. J. McGuigan (New York: Meredith Publishing Company, 1966).

70. Derrida, *Speech and Phenomena,* p. 77. Also cf. *Of Grammatology,* trans. Gayatri Chakravorty Spivak (Baltimore: Johns Hopkins University Press, 1976), p. 20. In such works, particularly the former, Derrida engages in an extensive critique of the notion that speech and the inner voice of thought attain the pure autoaffection of a transcendental mind, free of any embodiment. While attacking the transcendental phenomenology of Husserl, Derrida himself works with a phenomenology of the voice to understand the genesis of such notions. There is here an important convergence of Derrida's work with philosophers of the lived body, and in particular, with my own account. However, I would suggest that Derrida's primary focus upon textuality represents a new, though interestingly new, form of intellectualism, and hence remains open to a Merleau-Pontian critique.

71. It is precisely such abstract concepts that Havelock sees as largely confined to literate cultures. Oral cultures tend to physicalize principles through the figure of concrete human beings and actions, or other entities serving as agents ("The Orality of Socrates," p. 71).

72. Rorty, *Mirror of Nature,* p. 41.

73. Margaret Wilson, "Cartesian Dualism," in *Descartes: Critical and Interpretive Studies,* ed. Michael Hooker (Baltimore: Johns Hopkins University Press, 1978), p. 210.

Chapter Five: The Threatening Body

1. Regarding Plato, see Erik Nis Ostenfeld, *Forms, Matter and Mind* (The Hague: Martinus Nijhoff, 1982), p. 182.

2. Descartes, HR 1: 101.

3. Descartes, *Meditations,* HR 1: 190. Italics are mine.

4. Descartes, *Rules,* HR 1: 175.

5. Descartes, *Principles,* HR 1: 237.

6. Ibid., pp. 249–51.

7. Ibid., p. 251.

8. Descartes, *Meditations,* HR 1: 157.

9. Ibid., p. 198.

10. Ibid., p. 194.

11. Ibid.

12. Descartes, *Letters,* p. 111.

13. The full quote is as follows:

The body has an obstructive effect on the soul. We are aware of this phenomenon in ourselves, when we prick ourselves with a needle or some
sharp instrument: the effect is such that we cannot think of anything else.
It is the same with men who are half asleep: they can scarcely think of
more than one thing. In infancy, therefore, the mind was so swamped
inside the body, that it could think only of bodily matters. The body is
always a hindrance to the mind in its thinking, and this was especially
true in youth. (*Descartes' Conversation with Burman,* trans. and ed. John
Cottingham [Oxford: Clarendon Press, 1976], p. 8).

14. See, for example, Edwin Arthur Burtt, *The Metaphysical Foundations of
Modern Science* (Atlantic Highlands, N.J.: Humanities Press, 1952).

15. Descartes, *Meditations,* HR 1: 189.

16. Ibid.

17. Ibid., p. 145.

18. Descartes, *Conversation with Burman,* p. 8.

19. Descartes, *Letters,* p. 53.

20. Ibid., p. 233.

21. Merleau-Ponty, *The Visible and the Invisible,* p. 40.

22. Edmund Husserl, *The Crisis of European Sciences and Transcendental
Phenomenology,* trans. David Carr (Evanston, Ill.: Northwestern University
Press, 1970).

23. Merleau-Ponty, *Phenomenology of Perception,* pp. 383–88.

24. Thomas Kuhn, *The Structure of Scientific Revolutions* (Chicago: University of Chicago Press, 1962).

25. Patrick A. Heelan, *Space-perception and the Philosophy of Science.*

26. Descartes, *Passions,* HR 1: 344.

27. Ibid., p. 392.

28. Ibid.

29. Ibid. Cf. *Letters,* pp. 169–70, 173.

30. Descartes, *Letters,* p. 170.

31. Descartes, *Passions,* HR 1: 351–52.

32. Ibid., p. 352.

33. Ibid., p. 426.

34. Ibid., pp. 351–52. Also see John J. Blom, *Descartes: His Moral Philosophy
and Psychology* (New York: New York University Press, 1978), pp. 128–29 (Letter to Elizabeth, June 1645).

35. Descartes, *Passions,* HR 1: 355.

36. Ibid., p. 425.

37. Ibid., pp. 364, 406.

38. Descartes, *Letters,* p. 165.

39. See Heidegger, *Being and Time,* pp. 172–79; and Solomon, *The Passions.*

40*. As Jonas discusses (*The Phenomenon of Life,* pp. 99–102), far from being a secondary phenomenon, emotion is integral to, even definitive of animal sensorimotor life. Plant life is characterized by an immediacy of organismic fulfillment since the source of supply for metabolic needs is contiguous with the organs of intake. Such is not the case with animal life; its food stands apart from itself and must be pursued. Hence, it is necessary for animals to develop not only organs of locomotion and exteroception but an accompanying emotional life. The spatiotemporal distance between the start of pursuit and its fulfillment can only be bridged by a continuous appetitive intent. Directed long-range motility requires ongoing desires and emotions that motivate the chase for prey and the flight from predator. Otherwise the distantly perceived goal could not be sustained *as goal.*

41. Descartes, *Passions,* HR 1: 349–50.

42. Augustine, *City of God,* ed. David Knowles, trans. Henry Bettenson (Harmondsworth: Penguin Books, 1972), p. 577 (14. 16).

43*. In discussing the diagrammatic summation in chapter 4, I emphasized how dys-appearance typically reverses structures of disappearance, bringing to conscious awareness what previously was tacit. However, when the focus shifts from the question of personal awareness to that of personal control, a different structural possibility emerges. Within this context, disappearance and dys-appearance are often closely allied. That is, the withdrawal of a bodily function from the domain of the will (disappearance) can give rise to its experiential emergence as "Other" (dys-appearance).

44. Augustine, pp. 574–81 (14. 15–19).

45. See Blom, *Descartes: His Moral Philosophy and Psychology,* pp. 121–29, 143–48 (correspondence between Elizabeth and Descartes, May to September 1645).

46. Descartes, *Passions,* HR 1: 353.

47*. The moral condemnation of the body is a complex and multidimensional phenomenon that I will not seek to comprehensively delineate. I will only suggest that, in addition to the importance of dys-appearance in provoking this condemnation, disappearance also plays a role. For example, the body is often identified with the most immediate of physical cravings, such as for sexuality, pleasure, comfort, and food. Such corporeal desires are rightly seen as providing an inadequate foundation for a moral life. Yet what is thereby missed is the central role of the body vis-à-vis "higher pursuits," including spiritual practices, long-range goals, the giving of love and service, etc. For the body disappears from awareness in such ecstatically directed pursuits more than in those focused on immediate physical gratification, thus leading to the notion that virtue primarily belongs to the soul.

48*. Descartes, HR 1: 133. Cf. p. 141.

49. Ibid., p. 118.
50. Descartes, *Letters,* pp. 134–35. The quote is as follows:

I think I know very clearly that [souls] last longer than our bodies, and are destined by nature for pleasures and felicities much greater than those we enjoy in this world. Those who die pass to a sweeter and more tranquil life than ours; I cannot imagine otherwise. . . . And although religion teaches us much on this topic, I must confess a weakness in myself which is, I think, common to the majority of men. However much we wish to believe, and however much we think we do firmly believe all that religion teaches, we are not commonly so moved by it as when we are convinced by very evident natural reasons.

51. For a discussion of the importance of death in Descartes's *Discourse on Method,* see Ann Hartle, *Death and the Disinterested Spectator* (Albany: State University of New York Press, 1986), pp. 137–89.
52. Descartes, HR 1: 130.
53. Ibid., pp. 119–20.
54. Ibid.
55. In a 1630 letter to Mersenne, he regretfully concedes that he has not yet pursued the research into disease and remedies that would enable him to cure his friend's erysipelas (*Letters,* p. 9). Nine years later little has changed. Descartes writes to Mersenne that, though pursuing work on animal physiology: "I do not yet know enough to be able to heal even a fever. Because I claim to know only animal in general, which is not subject to fevers, and not yet man in particular, who is" (*Letters,* p. 64). Such admissions did not, however, stop Descartes from dispensing medical advice liberally to friends and acquaintances. See G. A. Lindeboom, *Descartes and Medicine* (Amsterdam: Rodopi, 1978), pp. 43–44.
56. Descartes, *Letters,* p. 184.
57. Descartes, *Philosophical Writings,* p. 314.
58. Descartes, *Letters,* p. 163.
59. Jack Rochford Vrooman, *René Descartes: A Biography* (New York: G. P. Putnam's Sons, 1970), p. 141 (5 October 1637).
60. Ibid., p. 142. The quotes are as follows:

I have never taken such pains to protect my health as now, and whereas I used to think that death might rob me of thirty or forty years at most, it could not now surprise me unless it threatened my hope of living for more than a hundred years. It seems very clear to me that if we would simply avoid certain things in our daily routine, we would be able to achieve a much longer old age than we do at present. (Letter to Huygens, 4 December 1637)

Since my profession now is largely one of timidity, and since I have gathered some knowledge of medicine, and since I feel alive and pamper myself with as much care as a rich man suffering from gout, it seems to me that I am at present farther from death than I was in my youth. If God does not grant me enough knowledge to avoid the ills which age brings, I hope that He will at least let me remain long enough in this life to have the time to bear them. (Letter to Huygens, 9 January 1639).

61. Ibid., p. 249.
62. Ibid., p. 246.
63. Descartes, *Meditations,* HR 1: 194–98.
64*. This methodological primacy of the pathological can introduce systematic bias into the sciences. Insofar as the animal is studied precisely at times when its functional synergies and world-relations are disrupted, an atomistic portrayal of embodiment is encouraged. (I later discuss this point in relation to the corpse.) For example, Merleau-Ponty argues that the reflex theory of animal behavior depends upon the artificial laboratory techniques employed:

> The reflex as it is defined in the classical conception does not represent the normal activity of the animal, but the reaction obtained from an organism when it is subjected to working as it were by means of detached parts, to responding not to complex *situations* but to isolated *stimuli.* Which is to say that it corresponds to the behavior of a sick organism— the primary effect of lesions being to break up the functional continuity of nerve tissues. (*The Structure of Behavior,* pp. 43–44)

Merleau-Ponty draws attention to what I have termed a motivated misreading, arising from the nature of dys-appearance. Episodes of natural and artificially-induced dysfunction, by bringing tacit mechanisms to the fore, provide a crucial tool for scientific investigators. Yet at the same time, such episodes motivate science toward misleading reductionist models; the "holistic" operations of the healthy body in its world are concealed by this concentration upon the pathological.

65. See Descartes, *Treatise of Man,* trans. and ed. Thomas Steele Hall (Cambridge: Harvard University Press, 1972), pp. xiii–iv.
66. See Plato *Cratylus* 400c, in *Collected Dialogues,* p. 437; and *Gorgias* 493a in *Collected Dialogues,* p. 275.
67. Margaret R. Miles, *Fullness of Life* (Philadelphia: Westminster Press, 1981), p. 14.
68. Descartes, *Reply to the Fifth Set of Objections,* HR 2: 210.
69. Descartes, *Letters,* p. 245.
70. Descartes, *Passions,* HR 1: 333.
71. Descartes *Treatise of Man,* p. 113. While Descartes is here referring to the hypothetical machine-analogue of the human body, it is clear that he means this as a description of human physiology.
72*. Descartes's notion of the body is far from univocal. As a number of authors have argued, Descartes also has an incipient theory of lived embodiment. See Spicker, *The Philosophy of the Body,* pp. 3–18; and C. A. van Peursen, *Body, Soul, Spirit: A Survey of the Body-Mind Problem* (London: Oxford University Press, 1966, pp. 18–33). For example, in his correspondence with Elizabeth, Descartes recognizes the intimacy of a mind-body union that, while knowable

only obscurely by the intellect, is immediately available to ordinary experience (*Letters*, p. 141). Zaner describes at length this "other Descartes," arguing that, in the face of Descartes's recognition of experiential mind-body unity, his employment of the machine metaphor for body was meant to serve only as a convenient fiction. See *Ethics and the Clinical Encounter* (Englewood Cliffs, N.J.: Prentice Hall, 1988), pp. 106–29.

I strongly agree with this recognition of the ambiguous and multivalent notion of embodiment operative in Descartes. While his physics and physiology demanded a certain rigorous notion of body as contrasted with the attributes of soul, he was too sensitive a psychologist and phenomenologist to disregard their union in the living person. He is thus led to ascribe functions such as perception not to *res extensa* or *res cogitans* proper but to a psychosomatic union that operates almost like a third substance within his philosophy. Descartes is thus not simply a "Cartesian dualist," but something more complex.

However, I would disagree with Zaner when he asserts that Descartes's comparison of the body to a machine is meant only as a self-conscious fiction. It is true that the body is not literally an automaton or clock. However, that the body operates just as a machine, that is, functioning according to mechanical principles, is precisely the grounding principle of Descartes's physiology. He does not see this as in any way challenged by the mind-body union uncovered in ordinary life, though we today might. The body-as-automaton remains his predominant model, and the one that has had the greatest cultural influence.

73. Carolyn Merchant, *The Death of Nature* (New York: Harper and Row, 1980).

74. Jonas, *The Phenomenon of Life*, p. 13.

75. Plato *Phaedo* 115c–e, in *Collected Dialogues*, p. 95.

76. Descartes, HR 1: 151 (italics mine). Though this statement represents his preliminary thinking prior to the application of metaphysical doubt, it is in congruence with his final views.

77*. This is not to claim that the corpse is merely one physical object among others, inert and neutral. Precisely as a lived-body-that-has-died, the corpse always retains resonances of ecstasis: hence, the medieval and early modern belief that cadavers could manifest certain sensorimotor powers, as well as sympathies and antipathies. See Philippe Aries, *The Hour of Our Death,* trans. Helen Weaver (New York: Alfred A. Knopf, 1981), pp. 353–61. It is only when decomposed, or dissected into organs, as in the case of Descartes's animals, that the sense of latent life is left behind.

78. Foucault, *The Birth of the Clinic,* pp. 124–48.

79. H. Tristram Engelhardt, Jr., *The Foundations of Bioethics* (New York: Oxford University Press, 1986), pp. 176–84.

80. Stanley Joel Reiser, *Medicine and the Reign of Technology* (Cambridge: Cambridge University Press, 1978), p. 30.

81. See Reiser for an ongoing discussion of this theme. Also see Eric J. Cassell, *The Healer's Art* (Cambridge: MIT Press, 1985); Richard M. Zaner, *Ethics and the Clinical Encounter;* Leder, "Medicine and Paradigms of Embodiment";

and Richard J. Baron, "An Introduction to Medical Phenomenology: I Can't Hear You While I'm Listening," *Annals of Internal Medicine* 103 (1985): 606–11.

82. Cf. Francis Barker, *The Tremulous Private Body* (London: Methuen, 1984), pp. 94–103.

Chapter Six: To Form One Body

1. Edmund Husserl, *Ideas: General Introduction to Pure Phenomenology*, trans. W. R. Boyce Gibson (New York: Collier Books, 1962), pp. 181–84, 191–93.

2. Don Ihde, *Existential Technics*, (Albany: State University of New York Press, 1983), pp. 42–44.

3. This paradox is reminiscent of that which Hegel describes of the "unhappy consciousness." Seeking to escape the animal functions, thought of as wretched and opposed to Spirit, this consciousness comes to focus ever more of its energy upon them. The sense of bondage to "the enemy" is paradoxically strengthened. See G. W. F. Hegel, *Phenomenology of Spirit*, trans. A. V. Miller (Oxford: Clarendon Press, 1977), pp. 135–36.

4. Wittgenstein, p. 48 (remark 115).

5. See Susan Griffin, *Woman and Nature* (New York: Harper and Row, 1978); Brian Easlea, *Witch-hunting, Magic and the New Philosophy: An Introduction to Debates of the Scientific Revolution 1450–1750* (Atlantic Highlands, N.J.: Humanities Press, 1980), pp. 241–52; and Janice McLane, "Controlling Nature, Controlling Woman: The Metaphysical Project of Mastery," Ph.D. dissertation, State University of New York at Stony Brook, 1988.

6. Easlea, *Witch-hunting*, pp. 236–38.

7. Peter Singer, *Animal Liberation: A New Ethics for Our Treatment of Animals* (New York: Random House, 1975), pp. 217–20.

8. Merchant, *The Death of Nature*, pp. 29–41.

9. Wing-tsit Chan, ed., *A Sourcebook in Chinese Philosophy*, p. 497.

10. Ibid., p. 530.

11. Wang Yang-ming, *Instructions for Practical Living and other Neo-Confucian Writings*, trans. and ed. Wing-tsit Chan (New York: Columbia University Press, 1963), p. 272.

12. Tu Wei-ming, *Confucian Thought: Selfhood as Creative Transformation* (Albany: State University of New York Press, 1985), p. 43.

13. Wang Yang-ming, *Instructions for Practical Living*, p. 222.

14. Tu Wei-ming, *Confucian Thought*, p. 47.

15. Ibid., pp. 70–73. Also see Julia Ching, *To Acquire Wisdom: The Way of Wang Yang-ming* (New York: Columbia University Press, 1970), pp. 52–74, 267.

16. Hwa Yol Jung, "Wang Yang-ming and Existential Phenomenology," *International Philosophical Quarterly* 5 (1965): 612–36.

17. Wang Yang-ming, *Instructions for Practical Living*, p. 257.

18. Ibid., p. 223.

19. Ibid., p. 273.

20. Ibid., p. 272.

21. Ibid., pp. 118–19.

22. Ibid., p. 273.

23. To speak of forming one body with the world is not meant to imply a denial of difference. My body is also that whereby I am localized and bounded, marked off as separate from other parts of the world. Yet it is precisely this divergence that allows for our connection. To perceive, I must inhabit a particular perspective and maintain some separation from the thing perceived. To live I must preserve a boundary across which I metabolically take in and give out. The "one body" relationship is thus a network of interconnection that does not obliterate the uniqueness of things.

24. Cf. David Michael Levin, *The Body's Recollection of Being* (London: Routledge and Kegan Paul, 1985), p. 151. In general, this work is a rich sourcebook for anyone interested in the question of embodiment. Moreover, Levin addresses in depth the aesthetic, moral, and spiritual import of the body— themes I will be discussing in this chapter.

25. In referring to the import of aesthetic and pragmatic concerns in evaluating interpretive vectors, I do not mean to dismiss the notion of truth. That is, I believe an ontology based on the notion of "forming one body" is true in a way that the Cartesian division of world into *res cogitans* and *res extensa* is not. However, to fully argue such a case, involving as it does a discussion of the nature of ontological truth, would take us far afield.

26. See Warren Thomas Reich, "Speaking of Suffering: A Moral Account of Compassion," *Soundings* 72 (1989): 83–108.

27. On shared celebration as a form of compassion, see Matthew Fox, *A Spirituality Named Compassion and the Healing of the Global Village, Humpty Dumpty and Us* (Minneapolis: Winston Press, 1979), pp. 3–4.

28. Max Scheler, *The Nature of Sympathy,* trans. Peter Heath (London: Routledge and Kegan Paul, 1954), pp. 14–18.

29. Fox, *A Spirituality Named Compassion,* p. 20.

30. Donald P. McNeill, Douglas A. Morrison, Henri J. M. Nouwen, *Compassion* (Garden City, N.J.: Doubleday, 1982), p. 16.

31. Whitall N. Perry, ed., *A Treasury of Traditional Wisdom* (San Francisco: Harper and Row, 1986), p. 598.

32. Wang Yang-ming, *Instructions for Practical Living,* p. 57.

33. Ibid., p. 273.

34. For discussion of the attitudes toward nature taken within the Western tradition, see, for example, John Passmore, *Man's Responsibility for Nature* (New York: Charles Scribner's Sons, 1974), pp. 3–40.

35. Stephen Clissold, ed., *The Wisdom of St. Francis and His Companions* (New York: New Directions Books, 1978), pp. 87–88. Compare Chief Seattle's statement, expressing a strong element of Native American spirituality: "We are part of the earth and it is part of us. The perfumed flowers are our sisters; the deer, the horse, the great eagle, these are our brothers. The rocky crests, the juices in the meadows, the body heat of the pony and man—all belong to the same family." As quoted in Fox, *A Spirituality Named Compassion,* p. 173.

36. For a discussion of the place of nature in Buber's work, see Donald L. Berry, *Mutuality: the Vision of Martin Buber* (Albany: State University of New York Press, 1985), pp. 1–38.

37. See Lynn White, Jr., "The Historical Roots of our Ecological Crisis," *Science* 155 (1967): 1203–7.

38. Martin Heidegger, *What is Called Thinking*, trans. J. Glenn Gray and Fred Wieck (New York: Harper and Row, 1968), pp. 14–15.

39. For discussions of the role of the body in traditional craftwork, as opposed to modern technological labor, see Levin, *The Body's Recollection of Being*, pp. 124–34; and Borgmann, *Technology and the Character of Contemporary Life*, pp. 40–48, 114–24.

40*. I have spoken as if compassion, absorption, and now, communion are separable dimensions of the life-world. To some extent they are. One would not confuse the experience of serving a sick friend with that of exulting in a forest's beauty or opening to the divine through religious practices. Yet such distinctions are also far from absolute. The modes of one-body relation mutually resonate and intertwine. Thus, felt communion mediated by spiritual practices may give rise to a flood of compassion. In the Judeo-Christian tradition love of God and love of neighbor are often seen as experientially inextricable. Likewise spiritual experience can be associated with aesthetic appreciation. Walking in the forest, we intuit the "glory of God's creation" or the "harmonious unfolding of the Tao." Then too, attention to the forest's beauty may awaken compassionate concern for its preservation. The moral, aesthetic, and spiritual dimensions are constantly intertwining, though one or another may dominate in a given person or at a given time.

41. See, for example, Charles Davis, *Body as Spirit* (New York: Seabury Press, 1977). For other works that address the embodied nature of spirituality, see John Y. Fenton, ed., *Theology and Body* (Philadelphia: Westminster Press, 1974); and Sam Keen, *To a Dancing God* (New York: Harper and Row, 1970).

42. Evan M. Zuesse, "Ritual," in *The Encyclopedia of Religion*, ed. Mircea Eliade (New York: Macmillan, 1987), 12: 406.

43. For this distinction, see Davis, *Body as Spirit*, pp. 22–24.

44. Shunryu Suzuki, *Zen Mind, Beginner's Mind*, ed. Trudy Dixon (New York: Weatherhill, 1970), p. 29.

45. As cited in Philip Kapleau, *The Three Pillars of Zen*, p. 205. The quotation is originally from *Zenrui No. 10*, an early Chinese Zen work, and is also to be found in Dogen's *Shobogenzo*.

46. Kapleau, *Three Pillars of Zen*, p. 268. I have omitted the author's numbering of her successive points.

Bibliography

Abram, David. "The Consequences of Literacy: Reflections in the Shadow of Plato's *Phaedrus.*" State University of New York at Stony Brook, 1986. Typescript.

———. "The Perceptual Implications of Gaia." *The Ecologist* 15 (1985): 96–103.

Aries, Philippe. *The Hour of Our Death.* Translated by Helen Weaver. New York: Alfred A. Knopf, 1981.

Aristotle. *The Basic Works of Aristotle.* Edited by Richard McKeon. New York: Random House, 1941.

———. "De Partibus Animalium." In *The Works of Aristotle.* Edited by J. A. Smith and W. D. Ross. London: Oxford University Press, 1912.

Augustine. *City of God.* Edited by David Knowles. Translated by Henry Bettenson. Harmondsworth: Penguin Books, 1972.

Bakan, David. *Disease, Pain, and Sacrifice.* Boston: Beacon Press, 1971.

Barker, Francis. *The Tremulous Private Body.* London: Methuen, 1984.

Baron, Richard J. "An Introduction to Medical Phenomenology: I Can't Hear You While I'm Listening." *Annals of Internal Medicine* 103 (1985): 606–11.

Basmajian, John V., ed. *Biofeedback: Principles and Practice for Clinicians.* 3d ed. Baltimore: Williams and Wilkins, 1989.

Berg, J. H. van den. "The Human Body and the Significance of Human Movement." *Philosophy and Phenomenological Research* 13 (1952): 159–83.

———. *The Psychology of the Sickbed.* Pittsburgh: Duquesne University Press, 1966.

Berry, Donald L. *Mutuality: The Vision of Martin Buber.* Albany: State University of New York Press, 1985.

Blacking, John, ed. *The Anthropology of the Body.* New York: Academic Press, 1978.

Blom, John J. *Descartes: His Moral Philosophy and Psychology.* New York: New York University Press, 1978.

Bordo, Susan. "Anorexia Nervosa: Psychopathology as the Crystallization of Culture." *The Philosophical Forum* 17 (1985–86): 73–104.

Borgmann, Albert. *Technology and the Character of Contemporary Life.* Chicago: University of Chicago Press, 1984.

Brener, Jasper. "Sensory and Perceptual Determinants of Voluntary Visceral Control." In *Biofeedback: Theory and Research.* Edited by Gary E. Schwartz and Jackson Beatty. New York: Academic Press, 1977.

Brentano, Franz. *Psychology From an Empirical Standpoint.* Edited by Oskar Kraus. Translated by Antos C. Rancurello, D. B. Terrell, and Linda L. McAlister. London: Routledge and Kegan Paul, 1973.

Burtt, Edwin Arthur. *The Metaphysical Foundations of Modern Science*. Atlantic Highlands, N.J.: Humanities Press, 1952.

Buytendijk, F. J. J. *Pain: Its Modes and Functions*. Translated by Eda O'Shiel. Chicago: University of Chicago Press, 1962.

———. *Prolegomena to an Anthropological Physiology*. Pittsburgh: Duquesne University Press, 1974.

Caplan, Arthur L., H. Tristram Engelhardt, Jr., and James J. McCartney, eds. *Concepts of Health and Disease*. Reading, Mass.: Addison-Wesley Publishing, 1981.

Casey, Edward S. *Remembering*. Bloomington: Indiana University Press, 1987.

Cassell, Eric. *The Healer's Art*. Cambridge: MIT Press, 1985.

Chan, Wing-tsit, ed. *A Sourcebook in Chinese Philosophy*. Princeton, N.J.: Princeton University Press, 1963.

Chernin, Kim. *The Obsession*. New York: Harper and Row, 1981.

Ching, Julia. *To Acquire Wisdom: The Way of Wang Yang-ming*. New York: Columbia University Press, 1970.

Clissold, Stephen, ed. *The Wisdom of St. Francis and His Companions*. New York: New Directions Books, 1978.

Daniel, Stephen L. "The Patient as Text: A Model of Clinical Hermeneutics." *Theoretical Medicine* 7 (1986): 195–210.

Davis, Charles. *Body as Spirit*. New York: Seabury Press, 1976.

de Beauvoir, Simone. *The Second Sex*. New York: Vintage Books, 1974.

Derrida, Jacques. *Of Grammatology*. Translated by Gayatri Chakravorty Spivak. Baltimore: Johns Hopkins University Press, 1973.

———. *Speech and Phenomena*. Translated by David B. Allison. Evanston, Ill.: Northwestern University Press, 1973.

Descartes, René. *Descartes' Conversation with Burman*. Translated and edited by John Cottingham. Oxford: Clarendon Press, 1976.

———. *Philosophical Letters*. Translated and edited by Anthony Kenny. Minneapolis: University of Minnesota Press, 1970.

———. *The Philosophical Works of Descartes*, Vols. 1 and 2. Edited by Elizabeth Haldane and G. R. T. Ross. Cambridge: Cambridge University Press, 1911.

———. *The Philosophical Writings of Descartes*. Translated by John Cottingham, Robert Stoothoff, and Dugald Murdoch. Cambridge: Cambridge University Press, 1985.

———. *Treatise of Man*. Translated and edited by Thomas Steele Hall. Cambridge: Harvard University Press, 1972.

Dickinson, Emily. *The Complete Poems of Emily Dickinson*. Edited by Thomas H. Johnson. Boston: Little, Brown and Co., 1960.

Dillon, Martin (M. C.). "Merleau-Ponty and the Reversibility Thesis." *Man and World* 16 (1983): 365–88.

———. *Merleau-Ponty's Ontology*. Bloomington: Indiana University Press, 1988.

Easlea, Brian. *Witch-hunting, Magic and the New Philosophy: An Introduction to Debates of the Scientific Revolution 1450–1750*. Atlantic Highlands, N.J.: Humanities Press, 1980.

Engelhardt, H. Tristram., Jr. "The Concepts of Health and Disease." In *Evaluation and Explanation in the Biomedical Sciences,* 1: 125–41. Edited by H. Tristram Engelhardt, Jr. and Stuart F. Spicker. Dordrecht: D. Reidel, 1975.

———. *The Foundations of Bioethics.* New York: Oxford University Press, 1986.

———. "Human Well-Being and Medicine: Some Basic Value-Judgments in the Biomedical Sciences." In *Science, Ethics and Medicine,* pp. 120–39. Edited by H. Tristram Engelhardt, Jr. and Daniel Callahan. Hastings: Institute of Society, Ethics and the Life Sciences, 1976.

———. "Illnesses, Diseases, and Sicknesses." In *The Humanity of the Ill,* pp. 142–56. Edited by Victor Kestenbaum. Knoxville: University of Tennessee Press, 1982.

Fenton, John Y., ed. *Theology and Body.* Philadelphia: Westminster Press, 1974.

Foucault, Michel. *The Birth of the Clinic.* Translated by A. M. Sheridan Smith. New York: Vintage Books, 1975.

———. *Discipline and Punish.* Translated by Alan Sheridan. New York: Vintage Books, 1979.

Fox, Matthew. *A Spirituality Named Compassion and the Healing of the Global Village, Humpty Dumpty and Us.* Minneapolis: Winston Press, 1979.

Freud, Sigmund. *Beyond the Pleasure Principle.* Translated and edited by James Strachey. New York: W. W. Norton, 1961.

———. *Civilization and its Discontents.* Translated and edited by James Strachey. New York: W. W. Norton, 1961.

———. *The Ego and the Id.* Edited by James Strachey. Translated by Joan Riviere. New York: W. W. Norton, 1960.

———. *Introductory Lectures on Psychoanalysis.* Translated by James Strachey. New York: W. W. Norton, 1966.

———. *Three Essays on the Theory of Sexuality.* Translated by James Strachey. New York: Basic Books, 1962.

Gadamer, Hans-Georg. *Truth and Method.* New York: Basic Books, 1957.

Gadow, Sally. "Body and Self: A Dialectic." In *The Humanity of the Ill,* pp. 92–99. Edited by Victor Kestenbaum. Knoxville: University of Tennessee Press, 1982.

Gorman, Warren. *Body Image and the Image of the Brain.* St. Louis: Warren H. Green, 1969.

Green, Elmer, and Alyce Green. *Beyond Biofeedback.* New York: Delacorte Press, 1977.

Griffin, Susan. *Woman and Nature.* New York: Harper and Row, 1978.

Griffith, Richard M. "Anthropodology: Man A-Foot." In *The Philosophy of the Body,* pp. 273–92. Edited by Stuart F. Spicker. Chicago: Quadrangle Books, 1970.

Guyton, Arthur C. *Textbook of Medical Physiology.* 7th ed. Philadelphia: W. B. Saunders, 1986.

Hartle, Ann. *Death and the Disinterested Spectator.* Albany: State University of New York Press, 1986.

Havelock, Eric A. "The Orality of Socrates and the Literacy of Plato: With

Some Reflections on the Historical Origins of Moral Philosophy in Europe." In *New Essays on Socrates*, pp. 67–93. Edited by Eugene Kelly. Washington, D.C.: University Press of America, 1985.

———. *Preface to Plato*. Cambridge: Harvard University Press, Belknap Press, 1963.

Heelan, Patrick A. *Space-perception and the Philosophy of Science*. Berkeley and Los Angeles: University of California Press, 1983.

Hegel, G. W. F. *Hegel's Philosophy of Nature*. Vol. 3. Translated by Michael John Perry. New York: Humanities Press, 1970.

———. *Phenomenology of Spirit*. Translated by A. V. Miller. Oxford: Clarendon Press, 1977.

Heidegger, Martin. *Being and Time*. Translated by John Macquarrie and Edward Robinson. New York: Harper and Row, 1962.

———. *What is Called Thinking*. Translated by J. Glenn Gray and Fred Wieck. New York: Harper and Row, 1968.

Heim, Michael. *Electric Language: A Philosophical Study of Word Processing*. New Haven, Conn.: Yale University Press, 1987.

Hume, David. *An Enquiry Concerning Human Understanding*. Edited by Eric Steinberg. Indianapolis: Hackett Publishing, 1977.

Husserl, Edmund. *The Crisis of European Sciences and Transcendental Phenomenology*. Translated by David Carr. Evanston, Ill.: Northwestern University Press, 1970.

———. *Ideas: General Introduction to Pure Phenomenology*. Translated by W. R. Boyce Gibson. New York: Collier Books, 1962.

———. *Ideen zu einer reinen Phänomenologie und phänomenologischen Philosophie*. Book 2. *Phänomenologische Untersuchungen zur Konstitution*. Edited by Marly Biemel, *Husserliana*. Vol. 4. The Hague: Martinus Nijhoff, 1952.

Hwa Yol Jung. "Wang Yang-ming and Existential Phenomenology." *International Philosophical Quarterly* 5 (1965): 612–36.

Ihde, Don. *Existential Technics*. Albany: State University of New York Press, 1983.

———. *Experimental Phenomenology*. New York: G. P. Putnam's Sons, 1977.

———. *Technics and Praxis*. Dordrecht: D. Reidel, 1979.

Jacobson, Edmund. "Electrical Measurements of Neuromuscular States During Mental Activities." *American Journal of Physiology* 97 (1931): 200–209.

Jonas, Hans. *The Phenomenon of Life*. Chicago: University of Chicago Press, 1966.

Kapleau, Philip, ed. *The Three Pillars of Zen*. Boston: Beacon Press, 1965.

Keen, Sam. *To a Dancing God*. New York: Harper and Row, 1970.

Kenny, Anthony. *Descartes: A Study of His Philosophy*. New York: Random House, 1968.

Kuhn, Thomas. *The Structure of Scientific Revolutions*. Chicago: University of Chicago Press, 1962.

Lacan, Jacques. *Ecrits*. Translated by Alan Sheridan. New York: W. W. Norton, 1977.

Langer, Susanne. *Philosophy in a New Key.* Cambridge: Harvard University Press, 1942.

Leder, Drew. "Clinical Interpretation: The Hermeneutics of Medicine." *Theoretical Medicine.* Forthcoming.

———. "Medicine and Paradigms of Embodiment." *The Journal of Medicine and Philosophy* 9 (1984): 29–43.

———. "The Rule of the Device: Borgmann's Philosophy of Technology." *Philosophy Today* 32 (1988): 17–29.

———. "Toward a Phenomenology of Pain." *The Review of Existential Psychology and Psychiatry* 19 (1984–85): 255–66.

Leibniz, Gottfried Wilhelm. "Monadology." In *Discourse on Metaphysics, Correspondence with Arnauld, Monadology.* Translated by George R. Montgomery. La Salle, Ill.: Open Court, 1980.

Levin, David Michael. *The Body's Recollection of Being.* London: Routledge and Kegan Paul, 1985.

Madison, Gary Brent. *The Phenomenology of Merleau-Ponty.* Athens: Ohio University Press, 1981.

McGuigan, F. J., ed. *Thinking: Studies of Covert Language Processes.* New York: Meredith Publishing, 1966.

McLane, Janice. "Controlling Nature, Controlling Woman: The Metaphysical Project of Mastery." Ph.D. dissertation. State University of New York at Stony Brook, 1988.

McNeill, Donald P., Douglas A. Morrison, and Henri J. M. Nouwen. *Compassion.* Garden City: Doubleday and Company, 1982.

Mahler, Margaret S., Fred Pine and Anni Bergman. *The Psychological Birth of the Human Infant.* New York: Basic Books, 1975.

Marcel, Gabriel. *Metaphysical Journal.* Translated by Bernard Wall. Chicago: Henry Regnery, 1952.

Margulis, Lynn and Dorion Sagan. *Microcosmos: Four Billion Years of Evolution from our Microbial Ancestors.* New York: Summit Books, 1986.

Marx, Karl. *The Economic and Philosophical Manuscripts of 1844.* Edited by Dirk J. Struik. New York: International Publishers, 1964.

Matson, Wallace I. "Why Isn't the Mind-Body Problem Ancient?" in *Mind, Matter and Method: Essays in Philosophy and Science in Honor of Herbert Feigl,* pp. 92–102. Edited by Paul Feyerabend and Grover Maxwell. Minneapolis: University of Minnesota Press, 1966.

Mattern, Ruth. "Descartes's Correspondence with Elizabeth: Concerning Both the Union and Distinction of Mind and Body." In *Descartes: Critical and Interpretive Studies,* pp. 212–22. Edited by Michael Hooker. Baltimore: Johns Hopkins University Press, 1978.

Merchant, Carolyn. *The Death of Nature.* San Francisco: Harper and Row, 1980.

Merleau-Ponty, Maurice. *Phenomenology of Perception.* Translated by Colin Smith. London: Routledge and Kegan Paul, 1962.

———. *The Primacy of Perception.* Edited by James M. Edie. Evanston, Ill.: Northwestern University Press, 1964.

_____. *Signs.* Translated by Richard C. McCleary. Evanston, Ill.: North-western University Press, 1964.

_____. *The Structure of Behavior.* Translated by Alden L. Fisher. Boston: Beacon Press, 1963.

_____. *The Visible and the Invisible.* Translated by Alphonso Lingus. Evanston, Ill.: Northwestern University Press, 1968.

Miller, Neal E. "Biofeedback and Visceral Learning." In *Biofeedback and Self-Control 1977/1978.* Edited by Johann Stoyva, Joe Kamiya, T. X. Barber, Neal E. Miller, and David Shapiro. New York: Aldine Publishing Company, 1979.

Mindell, Arnold. *Working with the Dreaming Body.* Boston: Routledge and Kegan Paul, 1985.

Norris, Patricia. "Biofeedback, Voluntary Control, and Human Potential." *Biofeedback and Self-Regulation* 11 (1986): 1–20.

Ostenfeld, Erik Nis. *Forms, Matter and Mind.* The Hague: Martinus Nijhoff, 1982.

Paivia, Allan. *Imagery and Verbal Processes.* New York: Holt, Rinehart and Winston, 1971.

Passmore, John. *Man's Responsibility for Nature.* New York: Charles Scribner's and Sons, 1974.

Pellegrino, Edmund D. "Being Ill and Being Healed." In *The Humanity of the Ill,* pp. 157–66. Edited by Victor Kestenbaum. Knoxville: University of Tennessee Press, 1982.

Perry, Whitall N., ed. *A Treasury of Traditional Wisdom.* San Francisco: Harper and Row, 1986.

Peursen, C. A. van. *Body, Soul, Spirit: A Survey of the Body-Mind Problem.* London: Oxford University Press, 1966.

Plato. *The Collected Dialogues.* Edited by Edith Hamilton and Huntington Cairns. Princeton, N.J.: Princeton University Press, 1961.

Plügge, Herbert. *Der Mensch und sein Leib.* Tubingen: Max Niemeyer Verlag, 1967.

_____. *Wohlbefinden und Missbefinden.* Tubingen: Max Niemeyer Verlag, 1962.

Polanyi, Michael. *Knowing and Being.* Edited by Marjorie Grene. Chicago: University of Chicago Press, 1969.

_____. *Personal Knowledge.* Chicago: University of Chicago Press, 1958.

Rawlinson, Mary C. "Medicine's Discourse and the Practice of Medicine." In *The Humanity of the Ill,* pp. 69–95. Edited by Victor Kestenbaum. Knoxville: University of Tennessee Press, 1982.

Reich, Warren Thomas. "Speaking of Suffering: A Moral Account of Compassion." *Soundings* 72 (1989): 83–108.

Reiser, Stanley Joel. *Medicine and the Reign of Technology.* Cambridge: Cambridge University Press, 1978.

Ricoeur, Paul. *Freedom and Nature: The Voluntary and the Involuntary.* Translated by Erazim Kohák. Evanston, Ill.: Northwestern University Press. 1966.

Rorty, Richard. *Philosophy and the Mirror of Nature.* Princeton, N.J.: Princeton University Press, 1979.

Russell, Bertrand. *Philosophy.* New York: W. W. Norton, 1927.

Ryle, Gilbert. *The Concept of Mind.* New York: Barnes and Noble, 1949.

Sacks, Oliver. *A Leg to Stand On.* New York: Harper and Row, 1984.

Sartre, Jean-Paul. *Being and Nothingness.* Translated by Hazel E. Barnes. New York: Washington Square Press, 1966.

Scarry, Elaine. *The Body in Pain.* New York: Oxford University Press, 1985.

Scheler, Max. *The Nature of Sympathy.* Translated by Peter Heath. London: Routledge and Kegan Paul, 1954.

Sherrington, Charles. *The Integrative Action of the Nervous System.* New Haven, Conn.: Yale University Press, 1947.

Singer, Peter. *Animal Liberation: A New Ethics for our Treatment of Animals.* New York: Random House, 1975.

Sokolowski, Robert. *Presence and Absence.* Bloomington: Indiana University Press, 1978.

Solomon, Robert C. *The Passions.* Notre Dame, Ind.: University of Notre Dame Press, 1983.

Spicker, Stuart, ed. *The Philosophy of the Body.* Chicago: Quadrangle Books, 1970.

Straus, Erwin. *Phenomenological Psychology.* Translated in part by Erling Eng. New York: Basic Books, 1966.

———. *The Primary World of Senses.* Translated by Jacob Needleman. Glencoe, N.Y.: The Free Press of Glencoe, 1963.

Suzuki, Shunryu. *Zen Mind, Beginner's Mind.* Edited by Trudy Dixon. New York: Weatherhill, 1970.

Szasz, Thomas S. *Pain and Pleasure.* New York: Basic Books, 1957.

Thomas, Lewis. *The Lives of a Cell.* New York: Bantam Books, 1974.

Tolstoy, Leo. *The Death of Ivan Ilych and Other Stories.* New York: New American Library, 1960.

Tondl, Ladislav. "On the Concept of 'Technology' and 'Technological Sciences.'" In *Contributions to a Philosophy of Technology.* Edited by Frederick Rapp. Dordrecht: D. Reidel, 1974.

Tu Wei-ming. *Confucian Thought: Selfhood as Creative Transformation.* Albany: State University of New York Press, 1985.

Updike, John. "Pain." *The New Republic.* 26 December 1983, p. 34.

Vrooman, Jack Rochford. *René Descartes: A Biography.* New York: G. P. Putnam's Sons, 1970.

Wang Yang-ming. "Inquiry on the Great Learning." In *A Sourcebook in Chinese Philosophy,* pp. 659–67. Translated and compiled by Wing-tsit Chan. Princeton, N.J.: Princeton University Press, 1963.

———. *Instructions for Practical Living and other Neo-Confucian Writings.* Translated and edited by Wing-tsit Chan. New York: Columbia University Press, 1963.

Welton, Donn. "Soft Smooth Hands: Husserl's Phenomenology of the Lived-Body." State University of New York at Stony Brook, 1986. Typescript.

Wertz, Richard W., and Dorothy C. Wertz. *Lying In: A History of Childbirth in America*. New York: Schocken Books, 1979.

White, J. C., and W. H. Sweet. *Pain: Its Mechanisms and Neurosurgical Control*. Springfield, Ill.: Charles C. Thomas, 1955.

White, Leonard, and Bernard Tursky, eds. *Clinical Biofeedback: Efficacy and Mechanisms*. New York: Guilford Press, 1982.

White, Lynn, Jr. "The Historical Roots of our Ecological Crisis." *Science* 155 (1967): 1203–7.

Wilson, Margaret D. "Cartesian Dualism." In *Descartes: Critical and Interpretive Studies,* pp. 197–211. Edited by Michael Hooker. Baltimore: Johns Hopkins University Press, 1978.

Winnicott, David. *The Family and Individual Development*. London: Tavistock Publications, 1965.

Wittgenstein, Ludwig. *Philosophical Investigations*. Translated by G. E. M. Anscombe. New York: Macmillan, 1953.

Young, Iris. "Pregnant Embodiment: Subjectivity and Alienation." *The Journal of Medicine and Philosophy* 9 (1984): 45–62.

_____. "Throwing Like a Girl: A Phenomenology of Feminine Bodily Comportment, Motility and Spatiality." *Human Studies* 3 (1980): 137–56.

Zaner, Richard. *The Context of Self*. Athens: Ohio University Press, 1981.

_____. *Ethics and the Clinical Encounter,* Englewood Cliffs, N.J.: Prentice-Hall, 1988.

_____. "The Other Descartes." In *Phenomenology and the Understanding of Human Destiny,* pp. 93–119. Edited by Stephen Skousgaard. Washington, D.C.: University Press of America, 1981.

Zuesse, Evan M. "Ritual." In *The Encyclopedia of Religion*. Edited by Mircea Eliade. New York: Macmillan, 1987. Volume 12, pp. 405–22.

Index

between, 119–25; as mind activity,
115–16. *See also* Mind;
Understanding, Descartes's concept of
Tolstoy, Leo, 83, 187n.2
Tondl, Ladislav, 179n.71
Tools, and incorporation, 33–35, 83–84
Touch: bodily absence in, 14–15, 17; as
motor activity, 17–19; sensory variety
in, 40–41; vision contrasted with, 118.
See also Hands
Treatise of Man, The (Descartes), 142, 143
Truth. *See* Epistemology
Tu Wei-ming, 157, 158

Uncertainty principle, 17
Unconscious: of Freud, 184n.35; of
Merleau-Ponty, 55. *See also* Recessive
body; Visceral body
Understanding, Descartes's concept of,
115, 119–21, 124–25. *See also* Thought
Updike, John, 74, 75

Visceral body, 36–68, 69; and depth
disappearance, 53–56; diagrammatic
representation of, 104–6; disease
contrasted with functioning of, 81;
dys-appearance by, 86–88; and
emotions, 136–37; indirection in
perception and control of, 49–53; and
Merleau-Ponty's concept of flesh, 62–
68; motility of, 45–49; perception by,
39–45; temporal depths of, 57–61. *See
also* Depth disappearance
Visibility and invisibility, Merleau-Ponty
on, 64, 67–68
Visible and the Invisible, The (Merleau-

Ponty), 2, 11, 62–68. *See also* Merleau-
Ponty, Maurice
Vision, 37, 41, 42, 87; background
attitude in, 24; and corporeal
background, 25; and dys-appearance
in disease, 85; invisibility of seeing to,
12–14, 25–27, 50, 113; as model for
mind concept, 117–19, 151; as motor
activity, 17, 20; "from and to" structure
of, 15–17. *See also* Eyes; Perception

Walking, hidden physiology of, 19–20
Wang Yang-ming, 149, 156–59, 161, 164,
167–68
"Western Inscription" (Chang Tsai), 156
White, J. C., 76
Whitehead, Alfred North, 68
Will, Descartes on, 129, 138. *See also*
"I can"
Wilson, Margaret, 125
Winnicott, David, 61
Wittgenstein, Ludwig, 154
Women: body consciousness of, 89, 98–
99; oppression of, 154–55. *See also*
Pregnancy
Writing, 122–24. *See also* Language
Wu-wei, 171

Yoga, 3, 56, 105, 153; control of inner
body through, 43, 52; and pain, 73
Young, Iris, 89–90, 190n.70

Zaner, Richard, 24, 93–95, 199n.72
Zen, 19, 29; beauty of commonplace in,
167; meditation in, 153, 170–72
Zuesse, Evan M., 168

Printed and bound by CPI Group (UK) Ltd, Croydon, CR0 4YY

09/06/2025

14685764-0001